MASTERING CHRONIC PAIN

Dr. Sahar Swidan
Dr. Matthew Bennett

Copyright © 2025 by Matthew Bennett & Sahar Swidan

ISBN(eBook): 979-8-9992580-0-7
ISBN(Paperback): 979-8-9992580-1-4
ISBN(Audiobook): 979-8-9992580-2-1

All rights reserved.

No part of this book may be reproduced in any form or by any electronic or mechanical means, including information storage and retrieval systems, without written permission from the author, except for the use of brief quotations in a book review.

Published by: TranscendMed

Cover Design by: Jane Dixon-Smith

Title Production by: The Bookwhisperer

To every patient who has ever felt dismissed, defeated, or defined by their pain—this book is for you.

May you find within these pages not only knowledge, but the fire to become your own fiercest advocate.

Not a passive sufferer, but a Warrior—someone who learns, questions, reclaims, and fights for a life beyond survival.

You are not broken. You are becoming.

And we are honored to walk this path of restoration with you.

And to our families—

whose steadfast love, patience, and belief made this work possible.

Thank you for holding space while we explored the complex terrain of pain, for understanding the late nights, the quiet obsessions, and the endless rewrites.

Your unwavering support gave us the strength to help others find theirs. This book is as much yours as it is ours.

With all our love, always.

BEYOND PAIN: A NEW PATH TO HEALING

Pain has a way of redefining a life. It narrows the world, dims its colors, and slowly rewrites the story we tell ourselves about who we are and what we are capable of. For years, the dominant approach to pain management followed a familiar script: a diagnosis, a prescription, and a hope—often unmet—that relief would follow. But as the opioid epidemic escalated into a national crisis, that script was abruptly torn apart.

By 2018, the devastating consequences of opioid overuse had become impossible to ignore. Overdose deaths soared, policymakers cracked down, and millions of people found themselves suddenly cut off from the only solutions they had ever been offered. The intent behind these restrictions was clear: to save lives. But for many living with chronic pain, the reality was a silent crisis of suffering—one in which doctors, untrained in alternative approaches, had little to offer beyond a sympathetic shrug.

This was the landscape in which *this book* was born.

Sahar Swidan and I had spent our careers deep in the world of chronic pain, not just treating symptoms but asking deeper questions—questions that most traditional medical training never prepared us for. Why do some people heal while others remain trapped in pain? Why do so many chronic pain patients suffer from fatigue, brain fog, and immune dysfunction? And most importantly: What if pain isn't just about the body?

We knew from our work in functional and metabolic medicine that pain isn't a problem of isolated parts—it's a full-body experience, shaped by nervous system dysregulation, inflammation, hormonal imbalances, and even the stories we tell ourselves about our suffering. We also knew something else: The traditional medical model wasn't equipped to address pain at this level. And so, in 2018, we gathered a team of experts and began writing a book designed to educate healthcare providers about these broader approaches. Ultimately, the book was published in 2021.

By then, the world had changed.

The pandemic shut down in-person learning. Conferences disappeared. Our book, meant to start a conversation among doctors, arrived in a world too distracted to listen. And while the need for a new conversation around pain had never been greater, we realized something even more important: We had been speaking to the wrong audience.

This book is our course correction.

We wrote this for *you*—not for doctors, not for researchers, but for the people living with pain every single day. We wrote it for the entrepreneurs, the athletes, the parents, the high performers who have tried everything and refuse to accept a life diminished by suffering. We wrote it for those who are ready to step beyond the outdated model of pain as a purely mechanical problem and into a new paradigm—one that treats the whole person, not just the symptoms.

This book is an invitation: to think differently about pain, to reclaim your agency, and to explore a path forward that is not just about reducing suffering, but about rediscovering resilience. We know the road isn't easy. But we also know that healing is possible—not just relief, but true, sustainable healing.

This is the beginning of that journey. Let's take it together.

— Dr. Matthew Bennett & Dr. Sahar Swidan

DISCLAIMER

The strategies these actionable chapters are designed to give you tools for improving resilience across the biopsychosocial model, but they are not a substitute for medical advice. Everyone's body responds differently, and it's important to discuss any significant changes with your healthcare provider before implementing them. While these chapters provide general guidance to help you explore what might work for you, your physician can help tailor these strategies to your individual needs. The strategies in these practical chapters are designed to support your resilience across the biopsychosocial model. But please remember: this book is not a substitute for medical advice and reading it does not establish a doctor–patient relationship with any of the authors.

Everyone's body is different. What works well for one person may not work—or may even cause harm—for another. This is especially true when it comes to medications or supplements, which can interact with existing conditions or prescriptions. If you're considering adding or adjusting any treatment, medication, or supplement, please consult with your healthcare provider first. They can help you evaluate what's safe, effective, and appropriate for your individual needs.

We've made every effort to provide well-researched, evidence-informed suggestions in these chapters, but they are meant as general guidance—not specific instructions. Your safety, context, and care plan should always come first.

INTRODUCTION

Sarah first felt the twinge in her lower back while reaching for a heavy bag of groceries. She assumed it would fade. But weeks passed, and the sharp, searing pain grew into something relentless.

She saw doctors, tried physical therapy, took medications. She followed every piece of advice she was given, waiting for the day she'd feel like herself again. But the pain didn't go away. It spread. What started as a discomfort in her back turned into stiffness in her legs, then deep exhaustion that no amount of rest could fix. It wasn't just her body anymore—it was her mind, her energy, her entire sense of self.

Sarah's world began to shrink.

She turned down invitations, unable to sit through a dinner out without fidgeting in pain. She started working remotely because long hours at her desk left her body aching for days. Her hobbies—the things that once made her feel alive—felt out of reach. Even conversations became exhausting; she found herself withdrawing from friends and family, tired of explaining what she was going through to people who couldn't understand.

The hardest part wasn't just the pain—it was the isolation.

One afternoon, while scrolling through old photos, Sarah saw a picture of herself hiking the Pacific Coast Trail with friends. She barely recognized the person in the photo. She used to be so active, so full of life. Now, she felt like a shadow of that woman, defined not by her passions but by her limitations.

A friend's question snapped her out of the spiral:

"What do you miss most about your life before the pain?"

Sarah had no answer. She had spent so much time fighting pain that she had lost sight of what she was fighting for.

That question planted a seed.

Instead of focusing on eliminating pain—a battle she felt she was losing—she started to ask a different question: What if I could rebuild my life alongside it?

THE BIOPSYCHOSOCIAL MODEL: A NEW WAY TO UNDERSTAND PAIN

For years, the medical approach to pain focused on the specific area of the body where the pain was felt—a sore back, a damaged joint, or an injured nerve. The question was simple: *What's wrong in this spot, and how do we fix it?*

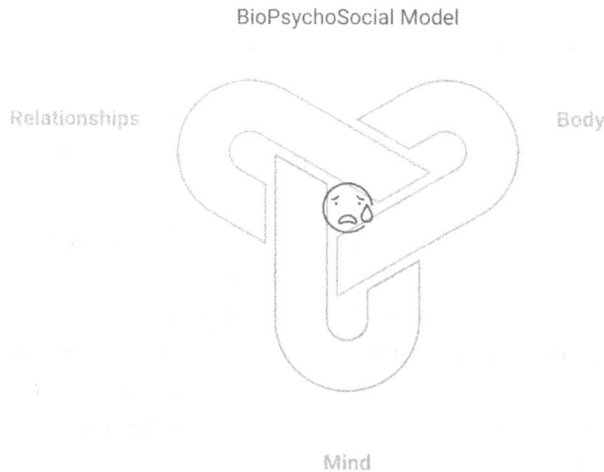

But chronic pain doesn't always follow this straightforward logic. Many people find that even after the injury heals, or despite a lack of clear physical damage, the pain persists. This has led researchers and clinicians to a profound realization: *Pain isn't just about what's wrong with the part of your body that hurts. It's about the systems that shape how your body, mind, and environment process that pain.*

But chronic pain doesn't just exist in the area that hurts—it can disrupt the very systems that are meant to keep you healthy and balanced. This is called **internal system sabotage**. It's a state where the body's systems—like the nervous, hormonal, and immune systems—become dysregulated, working against pain relief instead of promoting healing.

Here's how the biopsychosocial (BPS) dimensions contribute to this sabotage:

Biological Disruptions: Chronic pain sensitizes the nervous system like turning up the volume on pain signals. Studies on central sensitization have shown how the brain's pain-processing regions can become hyperactive, making even mild sensations feel overwhelming. This explains why chronic pain often persists long after an injury heals.

It can also throw off hormonal balance, flooding your body with stress hormones like cortisol.

It can keep the immune system in a state of constant inflammation. Elevated levels of inflammatory markers, such as cytokines, have been found in many chronic pain conditions. These markers can sustain the body's pain response, contributing to widespread discomfort and fatigue.

Psychological Factors: Anxiety, catastrophic thinking, or stress don't just affect how you feel—they can amplify your body's stress response, keeping your internal systems stuck in overdrive. Mindfulness practices have been shown to promote neuroplasticity, enabling the brain to rewire itself and reduce sensitivity to pain. This means that practices like deep breathing or meditation can do more than calm the mind—they can also physically change the way your brain processes pain.

Social Influences: Feelings of isolation or lack of support add another layer of stress, fueling the very responses that perpetuate pain. Research has shown that strong social connections can reduce stress hormones like cortisol, which are often elevated in people with chronic pain. This highlights the importance of rebuilding and maintaining supportive relationships as part of the healing process.

Together, these disruptions create feedback loops that keep the pain cycle alive.

THE PROBLEM: WHY CHRONIC PAIN FEELS INESCAPABLE

Chronic pain affects more than 50 million people in the United States alone, with millions more worldwide. It is the leading cause of long-term disability, yet for decades, treatment has been focused on one thing: symptom management. We've been taught to treat pain like a short-term problem, applying band-aid solutions instead of addressing its underlying complexity.

This approach isn't working. Medications provide temporary relief but come with side effects and risks of dependence. Surgeries can be life-changing for some, but they are invasive and don't always address the root cause. Even alternative approaches like physical therapy, acupuncture, or dietary changes—while valuable—don't work in isolation.

The reason is simple: chronic pain isn't just a biological issue. It's a *biopsychosocial* condition, meaning it is shaped by biology, psychology, and social environment. Pain alters brain function, disrupts the nervous system, and creates a self-perpetuating cycle of stress, fear, and avoidance. Healing must address all of these dimensions.

If you've ever been told your pain is "all in your head" or felt dismissed by doctors, family, or even yourself, you're not alone. Millions of people with chronic pain have been trapped in a medical system that doesn't fully understand them.

Chronic pain is a global epidemic. More than 20 percent of adults worldwide experience ongoing pain.¹ Of those, approximately 19.6 million say their pain is severe enough to significantly limit their daily activities—affecting work, relationships, and mental health.

Beyond the numbers are the untold stories of people who have seen their lives altered in ways they never imagined. People who have had to step back from careers they loved, turn down social invitations, or give up hobbies that once brought them joy.

Pain doesn't just hurt—it *reshapes your world*.

Many people with chronic pain describe a sense of losing themselves. They remember the version of themselves before the pain—the one who traveled, ran marathons, played with their kids without hesitation—and wonder if that person is gone forever.

If this resonates with you, know this: the problem isn't you—it's the way pain has been understood and treated.

THE SCIENCE: WHY PAIN FEELS SO RELENTLESS

As doctors who have worked for many years with patients navigating chronic pain, we've seen this story unfold countless times. The frustration. The exhaustion. The feeling of being dismissed. And we've seen what happens when people shift from fighting pain to rebuilding resilience.

Modern medicine is excellent at treating acute pain—the kind that results from injuries like a broken bone or a surgical procedure. But chronic pain is different. It isn't just a lingering symptom from an old injury or condition but an entirely different beast that changes the way the brain and nervous system function.

This is why treatments like painkillers, injections, and even surgeries often don't provide lasting relief. They target symptoms rather than root causes. Painkillers can provide short-term relief, but they don't address the overactive nervous system that keeps pain signals firing. Injections and procedures may dull certain areas of pain, but they don't

---

1. *The Lancet*, "Global Burden of Chronic Pain," *The Lancet* 395, no. 10225 (2020): 1013, https://doi.org/10.1016/S0140-6736(20)30345-9

INTRODUCTION

stop the brain from amplifying pain over time. Even physical therapy—while essential for some—can be ineffective if the brain is still locked in pain mode, interpreting every movement as a threat.

If you've tried these approaches and still feel like you're stuck in the same cycle, it's not your fault. Chronic pain is a whole-body condition that involves the brain, nervous system, immune system, and even emotions. And it can become a self-sustaining loop without us even realizing it.

First, the brain's pain system malfunctions. The brain becomes *hypersensitive* to pain, amplifying signals even when no injury is present.

Next, the body remains stuck in a prolonged "Fight or Flight" mode, unable to shift into its natural state of balance. Our autonomic nervous system (ANS) is designed to help us respond to threats and ensure our survival. Ideally, it operates like a well-tuned switch, shifting seamlessly between states of stress ("fight or flight") when danger arises and recovery ("rest and repair") once the threat has passed. However, chronic pain disrupts this system, trapping the ANS in a constant state of high alert. This prolonged activation leads to elevated stress hormones like cortisol and adrenaline flooding the body, which can increase inflammation, heighten pain sensitivity, and exhaust the body's natural resilience over time.

For example, imagine a person touching a hot stove—their nervous system immediately signals pain, triggering a quick reaction to pull their hand away, followed by a return to normal once the danger has passed. But with chronic pain, it's as if the nervous system keeps detecting the stove's heat even when the hand is nowhere near it, keeping the body in a state of tension and distress. This can result in symptoms like increased heart rate, shallow breathing, muscle tightness, and difficulty sleeping, all of which reinforce the cycle of pain and stress. Breaking this loop requires intentional strategies to signal safety to the body, allowing it to re-engage its natural healing and recovery processes.

When our autonomic nervous system (ANS) stops switching between stress and recovery modes, pain becomes more than just a symptom—it becomes a habit. The longer pain persists, the more the brain anticipates and reinforces it, like a well-worn path that deepens with every step. Over time, pain is no longer just a response to an injury or illness; it becomes something the body learns and expects, even in the absence of an immediate cause. This process, known as central sensitization, means that the nervous system becomes hypersensitive, amplifying pain signals and making even minor discomfort feel overwhelming.

Lastly, pain moves from affecting the body and brain to altering other aspects of one's life, including relationships and social connections. One of the most overlooked but devastating effects of chronic pain is the isolation it creates.

At first, you might cancel plans because you're having a bad pain day. Then, social gatherings start to feel exhausting—having to sit for long periods, explaining why you're not feeling well, or simply pretending to be okay when you're not. Over time, friends stop reaching out as often, not because they don't care, but because they don't know what to say. Family members grow frustrated or helpless, unsure of how to support you. Even in a room full of people, pain can feel profoundly lonely.

It's not just about missing events. Pain can change the way we relate to others. It can make you feel like a burden, or like your experience is too hard for others to understand. Some people with chronic pain begin withdrawing preemptively, avoiding social interaction to spare themselves the discomfort of being misunderstood. But this isolation has consequences—both emotionally and physically.

Research shows that loneliness can amplify pain. Social isolation increases stress hormones like cortisol, which in turn heightens inflammation and pain sensitivity. The brain, wired for connection, perceives loneliness as a form of distress, which can keep the nervous system locked in a state of high alert. In other words, the more disconnected you feel, the more deeply pain can take hold.

This is why addressing pain isn't just about physical healing—it's about rebuilding connection, too. Healing often starts with small steps: reaching out to a trusted friend, finding a support group, or simply letting yourself be seen and understood by others. Just as pain can reinforce itself in a cycle of stress and withdrawal, connection can create its own cycle—one of comfort, support, and resilience.

When we acknowledge that pain isn't just physical but deeply tied to our relationships and environment, we open the door to a different way of healing—one that doesn't just reduce pain but helps restore a sense of self.

The good news is that what has been learned, can also be *unlearned*. Through intentional interventions—such as retraining the nervous system with movement, breathwork, mindfulness, or cognitive reframing—the body can begin to rewrite its pain pathways. Just as the brain can form new habits in response to repeated experience, it can also build new neural patterns that signal safety instead of threat, gradually shifting the body out of its pain cycle and into a state of healing.

A NEW WAY FORWARD: YOUR BLUEPRINT THROUGH CHRONIC PAIN

What we've found as practitioners and experts in the chronic pain field is that the same mechanisms that make chronic pain feel inescapable are the same ones that make healing possible.

Just as pain can reshape the nervous system in ways that make it more sensitive, small, intentional changes can help rewire the brain and body toward healing.

This is where *resilience* begins.

If chronic pain is sustained by a web of disruptions across biological, psychological, and social dimensions, then healing isn't about finding one perfect solution—it's about creating a personal roadmap. This is where the idea of a Resilience Code comes in.

Just as every person's experience of pain is unique, so is the path to resilience. Your Resilience Code is built on identifying the systems in your life that are most affected by pain and taking deliberate steps to strengthen them.

Think of it like finding the weakest link in a chain. By strengthening that one link—biological, psychological, or social—that feels most disrupted, the entire chain becomes more resilient. This is often the system that feels the weakest, the one causing the most strain or imbalance.

For some, that might mean calming an overactive nervous system through relaxation techniques or better sleep (biological). For others, it could mean challenging negative thought patterns or addressing feelings of isolation (psychological and social).

The key is to start small. By strengthening one system, you create ripples of change that influence the others. Over time, this step-by-step approach builds a foundation of resilience that makes it easier to move forward. As the weakest of the links get strengthened, you are likely to find other weak links that were previously not recognized. Don't be surprised.

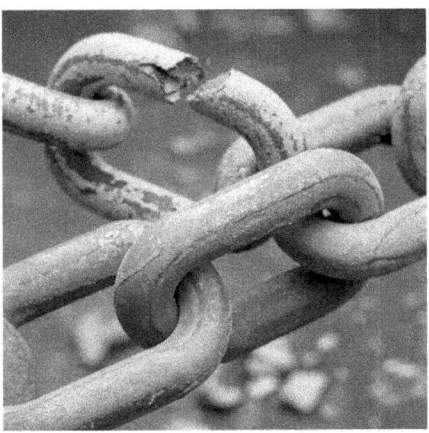

"What dimension of your life—biological, psychological, or social—feels the most disrupted right now? If you could focus on building resilience in that area, what small change would you try first?"

Your Resilience Code is unique to you. It's not a one-size-fits-all prescription or a rigid plan. Instead, it's a flexible framework that evolves as you uncover what works best for your body, mind, and relationships.

Throughout this book, we'll help you decode your pain by asking:

- Which area feels most impacted right now—biological, psychological, or social?
- What small, actionable step could you take to strengthen that area?

- How can you build on this progress to expand your resilience over time?

This approach isn't about fixing everything overnight. It's about creating a personalized strategy that works for you, allowing you to reclaim control, one piece at a time.

The beauty of the biopsychosocial model is that it empowers you to see the bigger picture while focusing on what matters most to you. By treating chronic pain as a whole-body experience and tailoring your approach to your specific needs, you gain the flexibility to address the areas that have the most impact.

This isn't about finding a quick fix. It's about building your resilience step by step, system by system, until the cycle of pain starts to loosen.

The biopsychosocial model allows us to approach pain in a way that respects its complexity and its solutions. It shifts the focus from simply "fixing" the pain to *healing the person.*

"When you think about your own experience of chronic pain, how might this broader view of pain help you better understand what's happening in your life? What part of this cycle feels most important to start with?"

Understanding how these disruptions occur is the first step to breaking the pain cycle. But knowledge alone isn't enough—you need tools to start applying this understanding to your life. Let's begin with exercises designed to help you identify where to start building resilience.

This book is for people like Sarah, and the many other patients who you'll meet in these pages. It's for people who have tried everything—medications, physical therapy, lifestyle changes—yet still feel stuck. It's for those who are exhausted by the cycle of hope and disappointment, searching for something more than temporary relief. It's for anyone who is ready to move beyond fighting pain head-on and start building

INTRODUCTION

resilience instead—a way to reclaim your body, your sense of self, and your future.

Here's how our journey will proceed:

Part One introduces the biopsychosocial model, which reveals how pain is an interconnected experience influenced by biology, emotions, and social connection. Through the stories of patients Emma and Maria, we'll explore how pain can shrink your world, making you feel isolated and powerless—but also how understanding how pain truly works can help you begin to reclaim control. Emma's pain nearly stole her identity as a passionate teacher, while Maria's injury threatened her lifelong career as a chef. Yet, each of them discovered that the key to resilience isn't just enduring pain—it's learning new ways to respond to it. These opening chapters lay the foundation for how pain rewires the brain and body, why conventional treatments often fall short, and how small, intentional changes can help you move forward. Pain doesn't have to be the end of your story. Understanding it is the first step toward rewriting it.

The first step in healing is understanding what's really happening in your body. Chronic pain isn't just prolonged acute pain—it rewires your nervous system, disrupts hormones, drains cellular energy, and fuels chronic inflammation. In **Part Two** how to break the pain-stress cycle and create a biological environment that supports healing. Through Lisa's journey, you'll see how breathwork, movement, sleep optimization, and nutrition can retrain the nervous system, restore energy, and calm inflammation. Healing isn't about suppressing pain—it's about rebuilding balance, one step at a time.

Pain isn't just a physical sensation—it's deeply influenced by emotions, thoughts, and learned patterns in the brain. Fear, stress, and negative thought loops reinforce pain pathways, creating a cycle that feels impossible to break. But through neuroplasticity, mindfulness, and cognitive reframing, you can train your brain to respond to pain differently. **Part Three** explores how chronic pain reshapes the brain—and how you can take advantage of neuroplasticity to reverse that process. You'll meet Andre, a former athlete whose battle with chronic pain forced him to rethink resilience, navigate, and come to terms with the fact that he had more trauma than he'd ever realized.

INTRODUCTION

Likewise, healing doesn't happen in isolation, as we'll see in **Part Four**. Chronic pain often leads to withdrawal, strained relationships, and loneliness—but connection is a key driver of resilience. The nervous system, immune system, and emotional well-being all respond to the quality of our relationships, making meaningful connection not just a luxury but **a biological necessity**. In this section, you'll explore how social resilience helps buffer the effects of stress and pain, and how to cultivate it in your own life. Through the story of Raj, who struggles with the isolation of chronic pain, and his wife Meera, who learns how to support him, you'll see how pain shapes relationships—and how relationships, in turn, shape pain.

Remember our primary message: Resilience isn't a one-size-fits-all solution—it's a personal blueprint, unique to you! **Part Five** will guide you in integrating everything you've learned into a structured, adaptable plan. You'll reflect on your progress, set realistic goals, and create a framework for maintaining long-term healing. Most importantly, you'll learn how to navigate setbacks with confidence, ensuring that resilience becomes a way of life rather than just a temporary effort.

Pain may be part of your story, but it doesn't have to define it.

Through small, consistent steps, you can retrain your nervous system, build resilience, and reclaim what pain has taken from you.

If you've been living with chronic pain, you might feel like you've lost a part of yourself—that the life you once had is out of reach. But resilience isn't about going back to who you were before pain; it's about building a stronger, more adaptable version of yourself moving forward.

This book is about reclaiming your life. Healing is not about perfection. It's about persistence, about learning how to move through pain rather than being consumed by it.

You are not broken. It is not all in your body or all in your head. Your pain is real, and it is everywhere. But your body and your mind are the most miraculous adaptable things. And with the right approach, you can find your way back to a life that is not defined by pain, but by possibility.

The journey towards resilience starts now.

PART ONE:
A PATH TOWARDS HOPE

CHAPTER 1
UNDERSTANDING PAIN IN YOUR BODY AND RECLAIMING YOUR LIFE

Emma had always been the kind of person who moved through life with purpose. Teaching social studies wasn't just her job—it was the heart of who she was. She loved the challenge of making history come alive for her high school students, the thrill of watching their eyes light up when they grasped a new idea. In her classroom, she wasn't just covering material; she was shaping young minds, helping students see the world—and themselves—more clearly.

She had always been a hands-on teacher. She moved around the room, gesturing animatedly, jotting notes on the board, flipping through textbooks as she answered questions. She stayed late to help struggling students, sat on the edge of desks as she discussed assignments, scrawled comments in the margins of essays with her favorite fine-tip pen. She was like one of those over-committed, big-hearted teachers you see in a movie, but she was real. Teaching wasn't just something Emma did—it was how she connected.

So, when the pain started, she ignored it.

It began as a dull ache in her wrists and fingers, creeping in after long days of grading. She chalked it up to overuse, the inevitable consequence of pouring herself into her work. But over the months, the ache turned into something sharper, a searing pain that flared when she wrote on the whiteboard or typed up lesson plans. Simple movements—holding a coffee cup, brushing her daughter's hair—sent electric shocks through her hands.

She told herself it was temporary. She switched to voice dictation software, asked students to help pass out papers, started wearing a brace at night. But the pain only grew worse, spreading up her arms, into her shoulders, settling deep into her body like an unwelcome guest that refused to leave.

One afternoon, in the middle of class, she reached for a textbook and felt her fingers go numb. The book slipped from her hands and hit the floor with a loud thud. Her students turned to look at her, their faces filled with concern. "Ms. Taylor?" one of them asked. "Are you okay?"

She forced a smile and bent to pick up the book. Then she panicked. Her hands wouldn't cooperate. She couldn't feel her fingers, couldn't get the muscles to cooperate with the simple act of scooping up a fallen book. A student rushed forward to help, and something in Emma's chest tightened. She had spent years being the strong one, the capable one. But now, in front of the very students she was supposed to be guiding, she felt small.

She felt weak.

That was the moment Emma knew: the pain wasn't just affecting her body anymore. It was stealing the part of her life that mattered most.

WHEN PAIN SHRINKS YOUR WORLD

After months of failed treatments—braces, physical therapy, anti-inflammatory medications—Emma's doctor suggested a surgery to remove stress on what he suspected was an impinged nerve. Desperate for relief, she agreed. The recovery was slow and grueling, but she clung to the hope that soon she'd be herself again. That she'd be able to return to the classroom, to her students, to the life she loved.

But even after the healing period, the pain remained. Different, but still there. Some days were better than others, but the unpredictability was exhausting. Would today be a good day, where she could type an email without flinching? Or would she wake up to a flare so bad she could barely button her shirt?

Her principal, once sympathetic, gently suggested a leave of absence. "Just until you're feeling better," they said. But all Emma heard was *You're not capable anymore.*

At home, things weren't much better. Her daughter, six years old and full of energy, wanted to play.

"Mommy, let's build a fort!" she'd say, tugging at Emma's sleeve. And Emma would have to force a smile, shake her head, say, "Not today, sweetheart." The disappointment in her daughter's face was like a knife in her gut.

Emma withdrew—from colleagues, from friends, even from her husband. It wasn't just the pain itself; it was the way it made her feel. For the first time in her life, she felt useless, powerless, broken. She was becoming a shadow of who she used to be.

One night, lying awake in bed, she found herself staring at the ceiling, wondering: *If I can't teach, if I can't use my body, if I can't be the mother and wife I used to be... then who am I?*

SMALL STEPS TOWARD HEALING

Scrolling through her phone in the dark, Emma came across a post from an old friend about mindfulness and pain management. She rolled her eyes. *How could breathing exercises fix this? My pain is real—not something I can just think my way out of.*

But the idea stuck with her. Over the next few days, she started researching how pain works. She learned about how chronic pain rewires the brain, making it more sensitive to pain signals. How stress and fear can amplify pain, keeping the nervous system locked in a state of high alert.

One phrase stood out to her: *Small changes make a difference.*

She wasn't ready to overhaul her life. But she could try something small.

She downloaded a guided meditation app and set a goal: five minutes a day of deep breathing. At first, it felt awkward. Her mind raced, and the pain seemed just as sharp as ever. But after a week, she noticed something: her worst time for pain—right before bed—didn't feel quite as unbearable. The sharpness dulled, just slightly.

Encouraged, she made another change. She reached out to a close friend, someone she'd been avoiding because she didn't want to explain how much she was struggling. They met for coffee, and for the first time in months, Emma laughed.

These weren't dramatic shifts. They didn't erase her pain. But they were the first cracks in the wall that pain had built around her life.

THE POWER OF RESILIENCE

Emma's story isn't unique. Pain doesn't just hurt—it isolates. It shrinks your world, making it feel like there's nothing left but the struggle to get through each day.

For Emma, teaching wasn't just a job—it was her mission. Standing in front of her students, inspiring them to think bigger, gave her a sense of purpose. But as pain spread through her wrists and arms, it began taking more than her physical abilities—it began stealing her confidence and her joy. The harder she tried to push through, the more pain pushed back, leaving her feeling like she was failing at the one thing that gave her life meaning.

That's the reality of chronic pain. It doesn't just hurt—it sidelines your passions, goals, and relationships, leaving you feeling isolated and stuck. Over time, the pain becomes more than a physical sensation. It shapes your thoughts, erodes your sense of identity, and shrinks your world.

But what science tells us—what Emma began to learn—is that pain isn't just something that happens *to* you. It's something your brain and body can adapt to. And just as pain reshapes the nervous system in ways that make it more sensitive, small intentional changes can help rewire it toward healing.

> **Key Takeaway:**
> Chronic pain doesn't just affect your body—it reshapes how you live and interact with the world. Recognizing this disruption is the first step toward rebuilding a life where pain doesn't define you.

SIDEBAR

Take Action: Reclaiming Connection

Pain thrives in isolation. But connection—to people, to purpose, to yourself—has the power to disrupt its grip.

Take a moment to reflect:

- What's one part of your life that pain has disrupted?
- What's one small step you could take to reconnect with that part of yourself?

Write it down. Make it real. And take that step.

Pain may be part of your story—but it doesn't have to be the whole story.

WHEN PAIN TAKES OVER YOUR MISSION

What Emma came to realize was that pain doesn't just live in your body—it seeps into your thoughts, emotions, and sense of purpose. It doesn't just cause discomfort; it rewires the way you interact with the world. It's a cruel, subtle wave that keeps washing over you until you've been silently removed from the things that . . . well . . . made you, you. As Emma found, the very things that once defined her, now felt like distant, inaccessible visions from another life.

At first, the changes are subtle. You miss a dinner with friends because the thought of sitting upright in a restaurant chair for two hours feels unbearable. You start turning down invitations for hikes, weekend trips, even short walks, not because you don't want to go, but because you're afraid of what the pain will do to you afterward. Maybe you keep pushing through at work, but the effort it takes leaves you drained and irritable, unable to enjoy the small moments that used to bring you joy.

For many, like Emma, chronic pain sidelines their mission—the part of life that gives them a sense of purpose and joy. Whether it's teaching, parenting, pursuing a dream career, or simply showing up for the people you love, pain makes you question your own capabilities. It isolates you, steals your confidence, and makes the world feel smaller.

Chronic pain doesn't just make movement difficult—it makes you feel like a shadow of who you used to be. But understanding this impact opens the door to something powerful: the chance to rebuild.

SIDEBAR

Take Action: Reclaiming a Small Piece of Your Mission

When pain takes over, it's easy to feel like everything is out of your control. But even in the midst of pain, there are ways to reconnect with what matters to you. The key is to start small.

- What's one small way you can reconnect with your mission?
    - Think about the part of your life or identity that chronic pain has affected most. Ask yourself:

1. What small action could you take today to re-engage with that part of your life?
   2. Could you write one page of a story you've been meaning to tell? Call a friend you've been avoiding? Spend five minutes doing something that used to bring you joy?
- Write it down and commit to trying it—even if it's just for a few minutes.

THE BODY'S SABOTAGE: WHY CHRONIC PAIN FEELS SO OVERWHELMING

Pain isn't just a physical sensation—it's a full-body experience. It affects your emotions, your relationships, even your ability to think clearly. And one of the reasons it feels so all-consuming is because of how deeply it's intertwined with the systems that govern your body and mind.

Think of your nervous system, your emotions, and your social world like a woven tapestry. When pain pulls on one thread, it ripples through the others, setting off a chain reaction that affects everything; likewise, when stress, isolation, or emotional distress pull at those threads, they can intensify your experience of pain.

Under normal circumstances, pain serves as a warning system. If you stub your toe or burn your hand, specialized nerve cells (nociceptors) send an urgent message up your spinal cord to your brain, triggering a response to pull away or protect the injured area. Once the damage heals, the pain fades.

But in chronic pain, this system malfunctions. Your nervous system becomes *hypersensitized*, meaning that even minor sensations—like a light touch, a change in temperature, or normal movement—can be misinterpreted as pain. It's as if the pain "volume knob" in your brain has been cranked up to maximum, making even mild discomfort feel unbearable.

This happens due to a process called *central sensitization*, where repeated pain signals cause the brain to reinforce and amplify the pain pathways over time. Neurons fire more easily, pain receptors become more sensitive, and even areas of the brain that normally regulate pain perception get caught in the loop, making it harder to dial things down.

For someone experiencing this, it can feel like their entire body is on high alert, as though they're constantly bracing for pain—even when there's no clear reason for it.

When pain becomes chronic, your body perceives it as an ongoing threat, triggering a prolonged *fight-or-flight response*. This is controlled by the *autonomic nervous system*, which governs involuntary functions like heart rate, digestion, and breathing.

During a short-term stress response—like narrowly avoiding a car accident—your body releases stress hormones like *cortisol and adrenaline* to prepare you for action. Your heart beats faster, your muscles tense, and your senses sharpen. In normal circumstances, once the danger passes, the system resets, and your body returns to baseline.

But with chronic pain, the stress never fully switches off. The body remains in a hypervigilant state, as if it's constantly expecting danger. This leads to:

- **Sleep disturbances.** You may feel exhausted but restless, waking up multiple times a night or struggling to fall asleep at all. Without proper sleep, your body loses its ability to repair and recover.
- **Increased muscle tension.** Many people with chronic pain carry tension in their shoulders, neck, and lower back without realizing it. Tight, rigid muscles can further exacerbate pain, creating a cycle of discomfort.
- **Digestive issues.** A prolonged stress response can slow digestion, leading to bloating, nausea, irritable bowel syndrome (IBS), or acid reflux.
- **Emotional exhaustion.** Being in a constant state of fight-or-flight can lead to increased anxiety, difficulty concentrating, and emotional burnout.

For people living with chronic pain, this isn't just an occasional stress response—it becomes a way of life. Over time, the body becomes depleted, struggling to regulate itself while pain remains ever-present.

Inflammation is the immune system's natural response to injury or infection. When you sprain an ankle, for example, your body sends out inflammatory chemicals like cytokines and prostaglandins to trigger swelling and pain—protecting the area while it heals.

But in chronic pain conditions, inflammation doesn't switch off the way it should. Instead of helping the body heal, it lingers, creating a state of low-grade, persistent inflammation that spreads beyond the original site of pain. This is often referred to as neuroinflammation, which is when inflamation spreads from the point of injury into the nerves themselves, further amplifying pain signals.

The effects of chronic inflammation can manifest in a variety of ways:

- **Widespread body aches and stiffness** that aren't linked to a specific injury.
- **Increased fatigue**, as the immune system continues to use energy fighting an invisible threat.
- **Brain fog and cognitive difficulties**, since inflammation can interfere with neurotransmitter function, affecting memory, concentration, and mood.
- **Heightened pain sensitivity**, as inflammatory chemicals further sensitize nerve endings, making pain more intense and widespread.

This ongoing immune activation means that even minor injuries, stressors, or infections can cause flare-ups, leaving people feeling as if they are constantly fighting their own bodies.

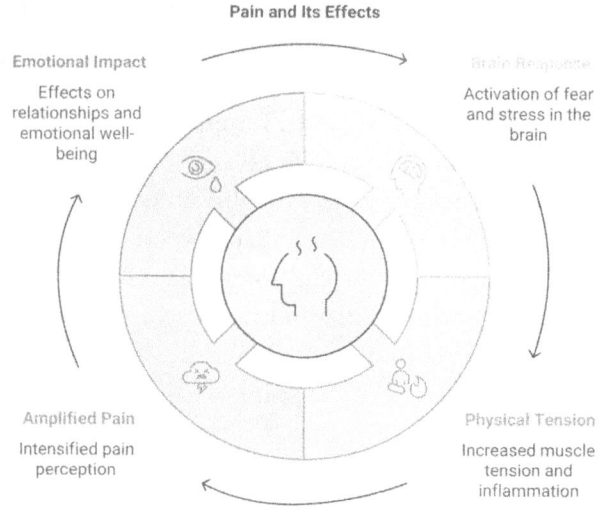

BREAKING THE CYCLE

Understanding how pain hijacks these systems is the first step toward breaking the cycle. By learning to calm the nervous system, regulate stress responses, and reduce inflammation, it's possible to retrain the body—helping it shift out of the "alarm" state and into a mode where healing can begin. It's possible to develop the resilience to navigate and begin reversing chronic pain through small, intentional steps, versus relying on the promise of medical-intervention-led "cures."

In the coming chapters, we'll explore how small, intentional changes can help reset these systems, making pain more manageable and giving you back a sense of control. We'll learn what Emma learned, small step after small step: that person you used to be, the one who feels like a distant shadow—they're still there.

We'll start this journey by first understanding the science of pain. What *is* actually happening in your brain, and your body, when something hurts?

CHAPTER-END AFFIRMATIONS

Reclaiming Strength, One Thought at a Time

Emma didn't wake up one morning and suddenly feel strong again. Healing didn't arrive as a single, dramatic moment—it was built through small, intentional steps. There were days she still felt lost, still questioned whether she would ever feel like herself again. But little by little, she began shifting how she spoke to herself. Instead of frustration, she tried to meet her body with understanding. Instead of measuring herself against what she *used to* be able to do, she focused on what was possible *now*.

Words matter. The way we talk to ourselves can reinforce pain's grip, or it can loosen it, creating space for hope, resilience, and self-compassion. These affirmations are not about ignoring pain or pretending it isn't there. They are about reminding yourself that *you are still here*. That you are more than what hurts. That even in difficulty, you are capable of joy, connection, and forward movement.

Read these affirmations aloud. Write them down. Let them be small reminders that, no matter where you are in your journey, you are not powerless.

- *Pain does not define me. I am more than what I feel in my body.*
- *Each day, I take small steps toward reclaiming the life I want to live.*
- *I honor my body's signals with compassion, not frustration.*
- *Even in pain, I can experience moments of joy, connection, and purpose.*
- *I am patient with myself. Healing is not about perfection—it's about persistence.*
- *I am not alone in this. I am worthy of support, understanding, and care.*

CHAPTER-END ACTIVITY

Recognizing Your Interwoven Pain Cycle

Pain isn't just physical—it seeps into your thoughts, your emotions, your relationships. It changes how you move through the world, how you interact with the people you love, how you see yourself. But just as pain can weave itself into every part of your life, so can healing. The first step is recognizing where pain has taken hold.

Take a moment to reflect on your own pain cycle. Grab a sheet of paper and draw three interconnected circles labeled Body, Mind, and Relationships.

In each circle, write down ways in which pain has affected you.

- Body: Poor sleep, fatigue, inflammation.
- Mind: Anxiety, brain fog, frustration.
- Relationships: Missed events, distance from loved ones.

Now, draw arrows between the circles to show how one area influences another.

- Example: Poor sleep (Body) → Irritability (Mind) → Withdrawal from loved ones (Relationships).

Emma's pain had taken her away from her students, her family, and, most of all, from the person she had once been. But the moment she realized this—truly saw it—was the moment she took her first step back. She didn't fix everything overnight. She simply noticed, acknowledged, and decided to do one thing differently.

Now, take a look at your circles. Where do you see patterns? Where has pain tightened its grip on your life?

Finally, ask yourself: What is one small action I can take today to interrupt this cycle?

It doesn't have to be big. Maybe it's texting a friend you've been avoiding. Maybe it's sitting outside for five minutes, breathing deeply.

Maybe it's taking a warm bath or stretching for a few minutes before bed.

Whatever it is, write it down. Commit to it. Let this be your first step—not toward erasing pain, but toward reclaiming the parts of your life that matter most.

CHAPTER 2
THE SCIENCE OF PAIN: WHAT'S REALLY HAPPENING HERE?

Maria had built her life in the kitchen. As the head chef of a bustling farm-to-table restaurant, she thrived on the heat, the precision, the rhythm of dinner service. She loved the way a well-run kitchen moved in harmony—pans sizzling, knives chopping, her team flowing through the space like a practiced orchestra. Food wasn't just her job; it was her identity.

Then, one evening, while lifting a heavy stockpot, she felt it—a sharp, searing pain in her lower back. She winced but kept moving. Kitchens didn't stop for minor injuries, and neither did she.

At first, she assumed it was just a strain. A few days of rest, some ice, maybe a heating pad, and she'd be fine. But the pain didn't fade. It deepened. It spread. Soon, standing for long hours became unbearable. The pain crept into her legs, radiating down like fire. Simple movements—bending to pull a pan from the oven, reaching to plate a dish—became moments of agony.

She pushed through, as she always had. But eventually, her body pushed back.

One night, mid-service, Maria turned to grab a sauté pan, and her legs buckled beneath her. She hit the tile floor hard, gasping. Her sous chef rushed to her side, but Maria barely heard him through the roaring in her ears. It wasn't just the pain—it was the realization that she couldn't do this anymore.

The doctor's orders were clear: rest, physical therapy, and time away from the kitchen. But rest wasn't in Maria's vocabulary. Who was she, if not a chef? What was left of her life without the adrenaline rush of service, the pride of running her own kitchen, the simple joy of creating something with her hands?

At first, she resisted. She convinced herself that she just needed to "fix" the pain. She cycled through treatments—painkillers, steroid injections, massage therapy. Some helped a little, but nothing lasted. The pain remained, an unwelcome shadow that followed her everywhere.

Her world began to shrink.

She stopped going to her restaurant, embarrassed to be seen struggling. She skipped out on nights with friends, too drained to keep up. Even cooking at home felt like a cruel joke. The kitchen—once her sanctuary—now felt like a battlefield she could no longer enter.

Maria had spent her career perfecting resilience in the kitchen. She could handle long hours, high stress, and impossible demands. But this? This wasn't just another challenge to push through. This was different.

And that terrified her.

WHY FIXING PAIN HEAD-ON DOESN'T WORK

As we've discussed, many people with chronic pain fall into the same trap: the belief that pain is a problem that can be *fixed*.

When we think about pain, we tend to imagine it as something temporary—an injury that heals, a signal that fades. And for acute pain, that's true. If you burn your hand on a hot pan, the pain is a warning system, a message to pull away. Once the burn heals, the pain stops.

But chronic pain doesn't work that way.

When pain becomes chronic, it stops being just a symptom of an injury and becomes something deeper—*a full-body experience*. The nervous system, brain, and immune system all become involved, reinforcing and amplifying pain signals, even after the original injury has healed.

This is why attacking pain *directly*—through medication, surgery, or even aggressive physical therapy—often doesn't work in the long run. It's like pressing harder on the gas pedal in a car that's stuck in the mud. The wheels spin faster, but the car doesn't move.

Instead, the key to breaking free from chronic pain lies in something deeper: *building resilience.*

After months of frustration, Maria reached a breaking point. She was sitting on her couch, phone in hand, absentmindedly scrolling through old photos. The images flicked past—plates of artfully arranged food, snapshots of her bustling restaurant, candid shots of her team laughing in the kitchen—but it wasn't until she landed on one particular picture that she felt something crack open inside her.

It was a photo from a year before the accident. She recognized the scene instantly: a Friday night rush, the kitchen in full swing. She was at the center of it all, sleeves rolled up, a towel slung over her shoulder, firelight from the gas burners reflecting in her eyes. Someone—she couldn't remember who—had caught her mid-laugh, a moment of joy stolen between the chaos. She looked *alive*. Focused, powerful, in command. She looked like *herself*—or at least, the version of herself she had once known.

Now, staring at that image, she felt an unfamiliar ache rising in her chest. Not just grief, but a sense of disorientation, as if she had stepped out of her own life and couldn't find the way back. She tried to remember the last time she had felt that way—strong, engaged, whole—but the memory wouldn't come. It had been lost somewhere in the months of doctor's visits, sleepless nights, canceled plans, and quiet, creeping withdrawal.

Had pain really taken all of that from her? Had she let it?

She looked away from the screen, her breath unsteady. The truth settled in her bones like a heavy weight: *I don't know who I am without the kitchen.*

It was that thought—not the pain itself, but the way it had stolen her sense of self—that undid her. She had spent so much time trying to *fix* her body, trying to force it back into working order, that she hadn't stopped to consider what else had been slipping away. Her connection to her craft, to the people she loved, to the small joys that had once anchored her in the world.

For the first time, she saw the real danger wasn't just the pain. It was what she would lose if she continued to wait—waiting to be healed, waiting to feel like herself again, waiting for a version of her life that might never return.

Something had to change.

She wasn't willing to let pain take everything.

So, after consulting with us, Maria made a choice. Her new approach, the one that we helped her build and hope to help you build as well, was a personalized blueprint meant to build resilience. The goal for Maria wasn't to *fight* pain, but to *rebuild her life around it*.

She started small, committing to three tiny steps that we suggested.

- Calming Her Body: Mornings were the hardest. She started each day with a 5-minute breathing exercise, focusing on deep, slow inhales and long, controlled exhales. At first, it felt ridiculous. But after a few weeks, she noticed a subtle shift—her body felt less tense, her mornings less overwhelming.
- Challenging Her Thoughts: Maria had always told herself, *If I can't work in a kitchen, I'm nothing.* She started to challenge that belief. Instead of fixating on what she *couldn't* do, she asked herself, *What can I still create?*
- Rebuilding Social Connection: She forced herself to reach out—to text an old friend, to invite her niece over to cook a meal together. At first, it felt forced. But little by little, these small moments reminded her that she *wasn't* alone.

None of these things "cured" her pain. But these small actions did something just as important: they gave her back a sense of control. And they gave her a foundation upon which to keeping building bigger and broader acts of resilience to reclaim her mind, her body, and her life from pain.

THE SCIENCE: HOW RESILIENCE REPAIRS THE BODY'S SYSTEMS

Resilience isn't just about pushing through adversity. It's a biological process—one that helps recalibrate the systems that chronic pain throws off balance. Resilience starts with the whole person. Chronic pain is not just a physical experience; it affects the nervous system, hormones, immune response, emotions, and even social relationships. A whole-person approach recognizes that pain is woven into multiple aspects of life—body, mind, and environment—and that healing requires addressing these interconnected systems rather than focusing solely on symptom relief.

When the body is in chronic pain, it often gets stuck in a state of imbalance—the nervous system becomes overactive, stress hormones surge, and the immune system can shift into a state of prolonged inflammation. Resilience acts as a counterbalance, helping restore equilibrium by calming the nervous system, stabilizing hormonal responses, and fostering psychological and social well-being. Instead of treating pain as an isolated issue, whole-person resilience focuses on strengthening the body's natural ability to heal and adapt, giving people a foundation upon which they can reclaim control over their lives.

Resilience isn't just about pushing through adversity. It's a biological process—one that helps recalibrate the systems that chronic pain throws off balance. Resilience starts with the whole person. Building biological resilience through the below focus points first helps calm these systems and restores balance.

Calming the Nervous System: Chronic pain keeps the nervous system stuck in *fight-or-flight* mode, flooding the body with stress hormones like cortisol and adrenaline. Practices like deep breathing, mindfulness, and gentle movement help signal safety to the brain, shifting the body back into a *rest-and-repair* state.

Regulating Hormones: Chronic pain disrupts the endocrine system, leading to imbalances in stress hormones. Resilience practices—like improving sleep, reducing stress, and fostering social connection—help regulate these hormones, reducing inflammation and stabilizing mood.

Reducing Inflammation: Chronic pain is often linked to low-grade, persistent inflammation in the body, which can amplify pain sensitivity and interfere with healing. When the immune system remains in a prolonged state of activation, inflammatory chemicals—like cytokines—continue to circulate, keeping pain receptors on high alert. Over time, this can lead to widespread body aches, stiffness, brain fog, and fatigue. Resilience-building strategies such as eating anti-inflammatory foods (like leafy greens, berries, and omega-3-rich fish), staying hydrated, prioritizing quality sleep, and managing stress levels can help regulate the immune response and support natural healing. Movement-based practices like gentle stretching or tai chi can also help reduce inflammation by improving circulation and supporting lymphatic drainage, allowing the body to clear out inflammatory byproducts more efficiently.

Strengthening Energy Systems: Pain drains energy—not just physically, but mentally and emotionally. Many people with chronic pain experience energy depletion at the cellular level, often due to mitochondrial dysfunction (the mitochondria being the "powerhouses" of cells that produce energy). Over time, pain-related fatigue can make even simple tasks feel overwhelming. Resilience practices help restore energy balance by slowly rebuilding the body's ability to produce and sustain energy. Small, consistent actions—like gentle exercise, restorative yoga, or even short exposure to natural sunlight—can support mitochondrial function and improve overall stamina. Nutrient-dense foods, proper hydration, and structured rest (as opposed to total inactivity) are also crucial for maintaining sustainable energy levels. The goal is not to push through exhaustion, but to nourish and rebuild the body's reserves over time, creating the foundation for greater resilience and movement toward an active, engaged life.

Reconnecting Socially: Isolation and loneliness are *biological stressors*. When people feel disconnected, the brain releases more stress hormones, which can increase pain sensitivity. After starting to get the nervous system, hormones, inflammation, and energy in check, by rebuilding relationships, resilience helps counteract this effect, releasing *oxytocin*, a hormone that promotes healing and reduces stress.

This is why resilience isn't just about *coping*—it's about *retraining the body to heal*.

Maria's journey wasn't linear. There were still bad days—days when the pain flared, when she felt like giving up. But she had a new way of thinking about those moments.

Instead of seeing setbacks as failures, she saw them as part of the process. Instead of trying to eliminate pain, she focused on *building a life around it*.

And slowly, something shifted.

She started cooking again—not in a restaurant, but in her own home. She experimented with new recipes, rediscovering the *joy* of creation. She taught small, private cooking classes, finding new ways to share her passion without the physical demands of a restaurant kitchen.

She wasn't the same chef she had been before. But she was still *Maria*.

YOUR PATH TO RESILIENCE

If you've been struggling with chronic pain, you might recognize parts of Maria's story (or of all the stories we've shared so far in these pages). Maybe you've felt like pain has stolen a part of you—your passions, your independence, your sense of self. Chances are you can relate. After all, you're here.

But here's what Maria's journey shows: *pain doesn't have to be the end of your story*.

The goal isn't just to reduce pain—it's to build a life that is *bigger* than pain. A life that includes joy, connection, and purpose.

So, ask yourself:

- What is one small step you could take today to *reclaim a part of yourself*?
- What's one belief about your pain that you could start to challenge?
- Who is one person you could reach out to, even in a small way?

Healing isn't about waiting for pain to disappear. It's about creating a life that makes room for both struggle and strength.

And resilience is the key. It's also a lifelong process, which can make it doubly hard to comprehend, embrace, and embody in a world where we're often sold quick fixes to complex problems.

Maria's journey didn't end the moment she decided to take her first step toward resilience. Neither will yours. This is, in fact, just the beginning of the work. There were still days when the pain flared, when she found herself longing for her old life in the kitchen. But there was a difference now—she had a strategy, a way to navigate the setbacks without losing herself completely.

One of the most important things to understand about resilience is that it's not a one-time fix. It's a skill—a practice—that evolves with you.

At first, Maria thought of resilience as something she needed to get through her pain, a bridge to a time when things might finally feel normal again. But as she kept going, she realized something deeper: resilience wasn't just a tool for dealing with pain. It was a way of living fully, no matter what.

She began to ask herself new questions:

- *What if resilience wasn't about getting back to who I was before pain, but about growing into someone new?*
- *What if I could build a life that made room for both struggle and joy?*
- *What if pain wasn't the enemy, but a teacher—showing me new ways to care for myself?*

Maria didn't wake up one day suddenly fixed. She knew that wasn't how her battle with pain was ever going to work. But she was learning empowered coping skills. She was learning how to recover from the hard days, and how to refocus on the parts of life that mattered most.

And that's the real power of resilience. It doesn't mean you'll never face setbacks. It means you'll have the tools to adapt, recover, and keep moving forward. And as you continue to grow, you'll discover that the life you're building is about much more than just escaping pain—it's about living a life that reflects your purpose.

SIDEBAR

Take Action: Living Fully Reflection Prompt

What does living fully mean to you? When you think about your own mission or passions, how might resilience help you reconnect with them?"

Take fifteen minutes to consider and then free write your response. Save these words. They will be a helpful light and a guide to which you can return throughout your journey.

HOW THE PEAK RESILIENCE METHOD WORKS

Building resilience isn't about sheer willpower. It's about learning where your systems are most disrupted—whether in your body, your thoughts, or your relationships—and taking small, consistent steps to restore balance.

The Peak Resilience Method isn't a one-size-fits-all solution. It's a framework that helps you identify your starting point and build resilience in a way that makes sense for you.

Unlike traditional pain treatments that focus solely on symptoms, this method helps address the underlying systems that sustain chronic pain.

The Peak Resilience Method

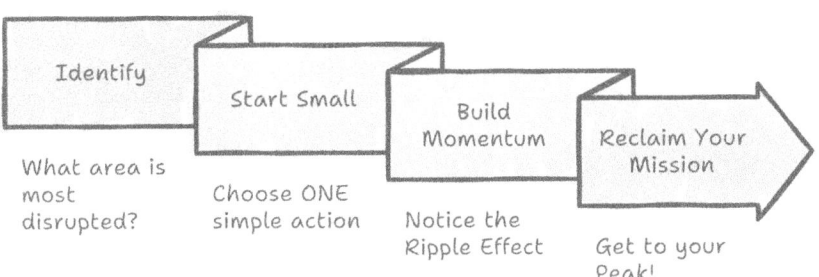

Think of resilience like a ripple effect. When you strengthen one area—whether it's calming your body, shifting your mindset, or rebuilding relationships—it creates changes in other areas, making it easier to break the chronic pain cycle.

The Peak Resilience Method helps you focus on the area of your life—biological, psychological, or social—that feels most disrupted. By taking small, intentional steps in that area, you can start rebuilding resilience from the inside out.

The Peak Resilience Method isn't just about coping—it's about creating a sustainable path to healing and growth.

It's based on scientific principles that have been shown to support resilience and reduce pain. Approaches like Mindfulness-Based Stress Reduction (MBSR) and Cognitive Behavioral Therapy (CBT) have demonstrated how targeted strategies can help:

- Calm the nervous system to reduce pain sensitivity.
- Reframe unhelpful thoughts that reinforce fear and stress.
- Strengthen social support to counteract isolation and emotional distress.

This book will guide you through these methods, helping you integrate the most effective elements into your personalized Resilience Blueprint.

By the end, you'll have a roadmap that aligns with your goals and empowers you to move beyond pain.

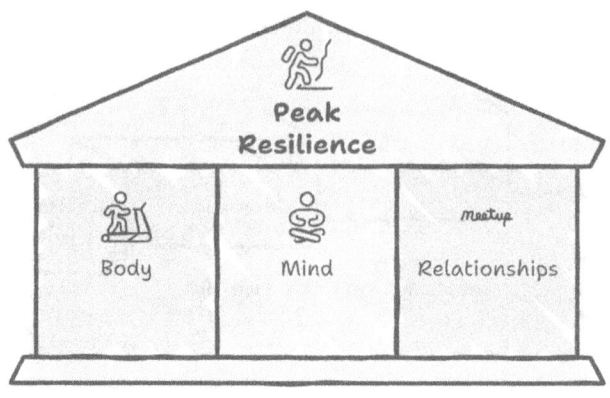

SIDEBAR

Taking Action: Three Small Steps to Build Resilience Today

If you're not sure where to begin, here are three simple actions you can take right now:

- **Biological Resilience:** Sit in a comfortable position and take five slow, deep breaths. Pay attention to the sensation of your breath as it moves in and out of your body.
- **Psychological Resilience:** Write down one thought that's been weighing on you and challenge it. Ask yourself, *What's a more helpful way to think about this?*
- **Social Resilience:** Text a friend or family member to let them know you're thinking of them. Connection can be as simple as starting a conversation.

> **Reflection Prompt**: *What is one area (biological, psychological, or social) where you feel confident? How could you use that strength to build resilience in another area?*

BUILDING A LIFE BIGGER THAN PAIN

Maria's journey didn't end with a single breakthrough moment. There was no dramatic turning point where everything clicked into place. Instead, resilience came to her in small, quiet steps—a morning breathing exercise, a shift in mindset, a simple meal shared with someone she loved. These weren't grand gestures, but they were enough to start pulling her life back from the grip of pain.

And that's the key to this process: resilience isn't about waiting for a cure—it's about reclaiming your life, one step at a time.

Like Maria, you don't need to have it all figured out today. You don't need to erase pain before you can start building something meaningful. What you need is a willingness to take small, intentional steps toward a life that feels more like your own.

Maybe that step is recognizing a belief about pain that's holding you back. Maybe it's reaching out to someone you've withdrawn from. Maybe it's allowing yourself to imagine a future where pain exists—but doesn't control you.

The path forward isn't about perfection. It's about persistence.

Maria's first step was finding small ways to soothe her nervous system—to quiet the constant stress response that chronic pain had wired into her body. This is the foundation of resilience: before we can rebuild, we have to create stability.

In the next chapter, we'll dive into biological resilience—exploring how chronic pain disrupts the body's natural balance and how we can start reversing that pattern. You'll learn practical tools to calm your nervous system, reduce inflammation, and create the conditions for healing.

Just as Maria discovered, resilience isn't just a mindset—it's something we build into our biology. And it starts with learning how to bring your body back to a place of calm.

CHAPTER-END AFFIRMATIONS

Rebuilding, One Small Step at a Time

Resilience is built in the smallest decisions—the decision to take one deep breath, to reframe one thought, to reach out instead of withdrawing. It's not about erasing pain but about reclaiming life, piece by piece.

These affirmations are here to remind you that even in uncertainty, even in struggle, you are building something new. You are more than what you've lost. You are capable of starting again.

Read these affirmations aloud. Write them down. Let them be a foundation you can return to, again and again.

- *I do not have to have all the answers to begin. I only need to take one small step.*
- *My identity is not limited to what I can or cannot do. I am whole, even as I change.*
- *Each moment of care—each deep breath, each act of kindness to myself—is a step toward healing.*
- *Setbacks do not erase my progress. Every day, I am learning new ways to live fully.*
- *My life is not on pause. Even now, I can find ways to connect, to create, and to find joy.*
- *I trust that with time, patience, and small, steady actions, I am building a life that is bigger than pain.*

CHAPTER-END ACTIVITY

The Peak Resilience Method in Action

Micro-actions, repeated over time, gave Maria back a sense of control and allowed her to start rebuilding her life around what was possible.

Now, it's your turn.

This activity is designed to help you take that first step in your own resilience journey. Rather than focusing on what feels overwhelming or out of reach, we'll identify where you already have strength and use that as a foundation to build on. Even the smallest shifts can create a ripple effect, influencing your body, mind, and relationships in ways that make pain more manageable.

Step 1: Pinpoint Your Strengths and Challenges

Instead of focusing solely on disruptions, this exercise helps you identify areas of strength you can build on.

On a piece of paper, draw three columns labeled **Body, Mind, and Relationships.**

Under each column, write:

- One area where you feel strong (e.g., *"I'm already consistent with gentle movement"*).
- One area where you're struggling (e.g., *"I avoid reaching out to friends"*).
- Circle the column where your strength could help offset your challenges.

Reflection Prompt: *"How can you use your existing strengths to start building resilience in areas where you feel less confident?"*

Step 2: Create a Micro-Step Plan

Big changes can feel overwhelming. The key to resilience is breaking actions into micro-steps that feel achievable and impactful.

Choose one action from the area you circled and make it smaller and more specific. For example:

- **Biological:** Instead of "exercise daily," commit to standing and stretching for 2 minutes after breakfast.
- **Psychological:** Instead of "journal every day," write down one sentence about how you're feeling.
- **Social:** Instead of "reconnect with friends," send a quick text to one person today.

Reflection Prompt: *"What's one micro-step you can take today that feels easy and doable? How will you measure success?"*

Step 3: Build Your Momentum Tracker

Tracking small wins helps reinforce progress and motivation over time. You can create a "Momentum Tracker" using a simple grid.

Day: Write the date.
Action: Record one resilience-building action you took that day.
Result: Reflect briefly on how it felt or what changed.

Day	Action	Result

At the end of the week, review your tracker and ask:

- *"What patterns am I noticing?"*
- *"Where am I seeing the biggest shifts?"*

If a formal tracker feels overwhelming, try a simpler approach: at the end of each day, take 30 seconds to reflect on one thing you did to support your resilience. No need to write it down—just take a moment to notice the progress you're making.

Reflection Prompt: *Imagine what's possible when pain no longer defines you. What could you accomplish? How could you live if your life was centered not on pain, but on passion and purpose? The journey won't always be easy. But every step you take brings you closer to a life that reflects who you truly are.*

PART TWO:
BIOLOGICAL RESILIENCE – REWIRING THE BODY

CHAPTER 3
RECLAIMING STABILITY IN YOUR BIOLOGICAL SYSTEMS

Lisa had always considered herself strong. As a mother of two, she prided herself on keeping up with her kids, managing her job, and making time for family dinners. But over the years, chronic back pain had chipped away at that strength. What had started as an occasional discomfort turned into an unrelenting ache that dictated the pace of her life.

Mornings were the worst. She would wake up stiff, her lower back feeling as if it had been welded in place overnight. Lifting her toddler sent bolts of pain shooting down her spine. By mid-afternoon, just sitting through a work meeting left her exhausted. She had tried everything—painkillers, physical therapy, hot and cold packs—but nothing seemed to provide lasting relief.

At one point, her doctor suggested looking at her biological resilience—how her body's internal systems were managing pain and stress. Lisa had rolled her eyes at the idea. *How could something like my diet or my sleep really change my pain?* she had thought. But after years of frustration, she was willing to try something different.

Lisa's journey wasn't about quick fixes. It was about learning how chronic pain disrupts the body's delicate balance—and how small, intentional changes could begin to restore that balance.

Pain isn't just about the nerves—it's about the entire body. Chronic pain doesn't just linger at the site of an old injury; it spreads into the nervous system, immune system, endocrine system, and even the body's cellular energy production.

Lisa had never considered this before. Like many people, she had thought of pain as a localized problem—an issue with her back. But as she started learning, she began to see how *biological resilience* was about more than just pain management. It was about restoring balance in her body's internal systems so they could function as they were meant to.

She started to wonder—why wasn't her pain going away? Why did she feel exhausted all the time? Why did small stressors make her pain worse? It turns out, pain wasn't just disrupting one part of her body—it was affecting everything.

HOW DOES INTERNAL SYSTEM SABOTAGE HAPPEN?

You've already learned that chronic pain isn't just a lingering signal from an injury—it's a whole-body experience. In this chapter, we'll dive deeper into the biological systems that can become disrupted in chronic pain: the nervous, endocrine, and immune systems. These systems work together to protect you, but in chronic pain, they can fall out of sync, creating feedback loops that sustain pain rather than resolve it.

Pain doesn't always start with a traumatic injury. Sometimes, severe or prolonged pain from an illness or minor injury can cause these systems to malfunction. But it's also possible for this dysfunction to develop without a clear physical cause, setting the stage for chronic pain.

The body's biological systems are designed to adapt to stress and recover. But when stressors are severe, prolonged, or layered over time, these systems can become stuck in patterns that perpetuate pain and dysfunction. Factors that contribute to this include:

Stressful Life Events: Chronic stress, trauma, or emotional upheaval can push the nervous system into a prolonged "fight or flight" state, even in the absence of physical injury.

For example, someone experiencing years of workplace stress or caregiving burnout might develop physical pain rooted in biological dysregulation.

Sleep Deprivation or Poor Sleep Quality: Sleep is crucial for restoring balance in the nervous, endocrine, and immune systems. Poor sleep disrupts the body's natural repair processes, making it harder to recover from pain.

Diet and Gut Health: A diet high in processed foods, sugar, and unhealthy fats can promote chronic inflammation, which sensitizes nerves and exacerbates pain. Imbalances in gut health—caused by stress, poor diet, or illness—can lead to an overactive immune response and heightened pain sensitivity. In chapter six, we'll explore the full gut-brain connection.

Hormonal Changes or Imbalances: Conditions like chronic stress or hormonal shifts (e.g., menopause, thyroid dysfunction) can amplify pain and disrupt resilience.

Genetics and Past Experiences: Some individuals may have a genetic predisposition to nervous system hypersensitivity or a history of adverse childhood experiences (ACEs), both of which can increase the likelihood of chronic pain. We'll look more at the role of trauma in chapter eight.

While internal system sabotage may sound overwhelming, it's important to remember that these patterns are not permanent. The body has an incredible capacity to heal and adapt when given the right support.

In this and the next chapter, we'll explore the primary bodily systems impacted by chronic pain:

1. **The nervous system** and how calming its hypersensitivity can reduce pain.
2. **The endocrine system**, and how balancing stress hormones can improve sleep and healing.
3. **The immune system**, and how calming inflammation supports recovery.
4. **The mitochondrial energy system** and how improving cellular energy production can restore vitality and reduce fatigue.

Each of these systems plays a role in keeping chronic pain alive, but each also holds opportunities for healing. By addressing one system, you can create a ripple effect that strengthens the others, helping you break the pain cycle and reclaim control.

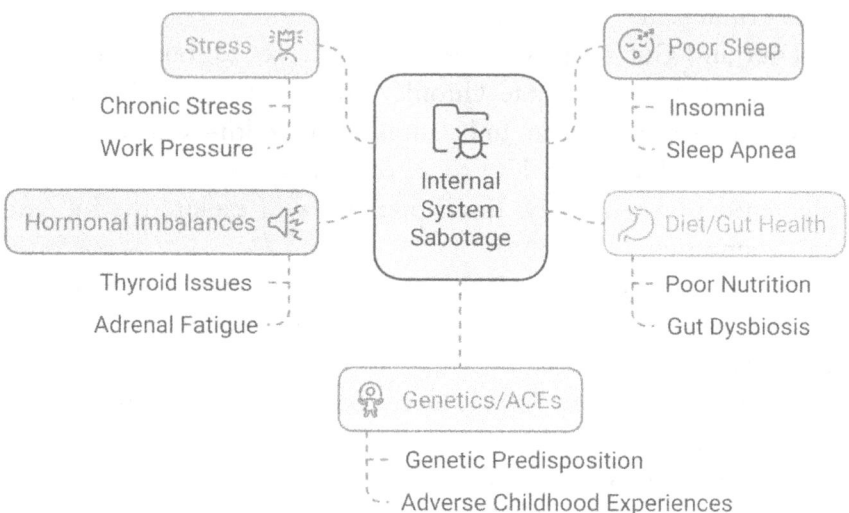

THE NERVOUS SYSTEM: OVERLOAD AND SENSITIZATION

Lisa sat in her car outside the grocery store, gripping the steering wheel with white-knuckled tension. The pain in her lower back pulsed like a warning light, an ever-present reminder of her body's betrayal. She had spent the last ten minutes debating whether she had the energy to walk the aisles, grab a few essentials, and make it home without collapsing in exhaustion.

It wasn't just about the physical pain anymore—it was the exhaustion of anticipating it. The fear of a sudden flare-up, the way her body tensed at the thought of another sleepless night, the quiet dread that had settled over her daily life. Her nervous system felt like a wire stretched too thin, vibrating with an invisible current of stress.

She didn't know it yet, but what she was experiencing wasn't just about her injured back. Her nervous system had rewired itself in response to chronic pain, turning her body into a hypervigilant alarm system, always on edge, always expecting the worst.

The Science of Sensitization: Turning Up the Volume

Your nervous system is your body's command center. It governs everything from movement and reflexes to thoughts and emotions. At its core, the nervous system functions as a vast communication network, sending electrical and chemical signals throughout the body to help it respond to the world.

Pain is one of the body's most primal defense mechanisms. When you stub your toe or burn your hand, pain signals travel from specialized nerve cells (nociceptors) up the spinal cord to the brain, where they trigger a response: pull away, protect, heal. In an ideal system, once the danger has passed, the pain fades, and the body resets.

But in chronic pain, something goes wrong. The nervous system doesn't turn off the alarm—it keeps the volume cranked up, long after the initial injury has healed. This phenomenon, called sensitization, is at the root of why chronic pain feels so overwhelming.

Neuroscientists have spent decades studying why chronic pain persists, and the concept of central sensitization has emerged as a key explanation. When pain is prolonged, the central nervous system—particularly the spinal cord and brain—becomes hypersensitive, amplifying pain signals even when there is no ongoing tissue damage.

Think of it like this: imagine a house alarm that was triggered by a break-in. Normally, once the intruder is gone, the system resets. But with central sensitization, the alarm stays on permanently—not just blaring at actual threats, but also reacting to harmless movements, light touches, or even stress and emotions.

Studies in pain neuroscience have shown that people with chronic pain experience heightened activity in the brain's pain-processing regions, such as the anterior cingulate cortex, insula, and amygdala. Over time, these regions reinforce pain pathways, making the nervous system even more efficient at producing pain—regardless of physical injury.

One of the earliest clues to this phenomenon came from amputee patients who experienced phantom limb pain—searing pain in a limb that no longer existed. In the 1990s, neuroscientist V.S. Ramachandran discovered that the brain had "mapped" the missing limb so thoroughly that it continued generating pain signals despite the limb's absence. This revealed a key truth: pain is not just in the body—it is in the brain.

This concept led to the field of neuroplasticity, the brain's ability to reorganize itself based on experience. Just as the brain can learn pain, it can also unlearn it.

For Lisa, this meant that her pain wasn't just coming from her back—it was coming from a nervous system that had learned pain too well. And if her nervous system could learn pain, it could also learn something new.

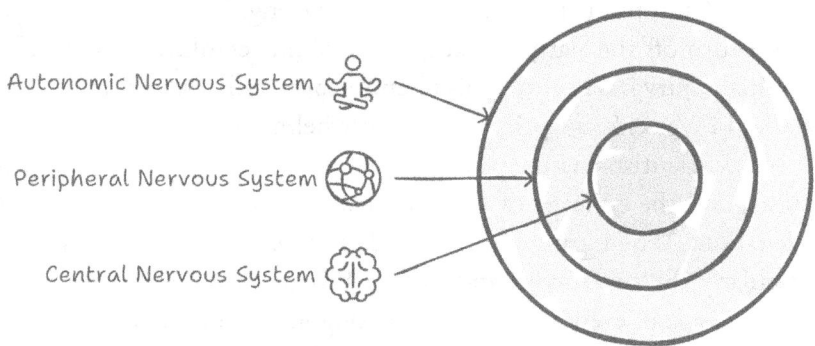

Breaking the Cycle: Calming an Overactive Nervous System

Understanding that her pain was being amplified by a hypersensitive nervous system was both frustrating and liberating. It meant that no single surgery or pill would "fix" her—but it also meant that she had a way forward. She could train her nervous system to stop sounding the alarm.

Her first step was breathwork.

Her physical therapist suggested a simple exercise: diaphragmatic breathing, also called parasympathetic breathing.

"Your nervous system has two main settings: fight-or-flight and rest-and-repair," her therapist explained. "Chronic pain keeps you stuck in fight-or-flight. But deep, slow breathing signals to your brain that you're safe. It helps shift your nervous system into rest-and-repair mode, which is where healing happens."

Skeptical but willing to try, Lisa began practicing for two minutes each morning and evening. She inhaled deeply through her nose, feeling her belly rise, then exhaled slowly through pursed lips. At first, it felt unnatural. But by the end of the week, she noticed something unexpected: her pain wasn't gone, but her body felt less tense.

This was her first real proof that she could influence her nervous system.

For Lisa, learning to work with her nervous system instead of against it became a turning point. She wasn't just managing pain—she was reshaping how her body experienced it.

She had spent years believing that pain was something that happened to her. Now, she was realizing she had a say in how her nervous system responded.

And that changed everything.

SIDEBAR

Taking Action: Retraining Your Nervous System

You may not even realize this is happening to you. The signs can be easy to miss and the slide into pain a subtle build. But if your nervous system has become hypersensitive to pain, one of the most effective ways to calm it is to engage the parasympathetic nervous system—the body's natural counterbalance to stress.

Try this five-minute nervous system reset:

1. Find a Quiet Space – Sit or lie down in a comfortable position. Close your eyes if it feels safe.
2. Diaphragmatic Breathing – Place one hand on your belly. Inhale deeply through your nose for a count of 4, expanding your belly. Hold for 4 seconds. Exhale slowly through pursed lips for 6 seconds. Repeat 5 times.
3. Progressive Relaxation – Starting at your feet, tense your muscles for 5 seconds, then release. Move upward, relaxing your legs, shoulders, and jaw.
4. Visualize Safety – Imagine a place where you feel completely safe and at ease—a cozy cabin, a quiet beach, a childhood home. Let yourself feel what it's like to be safe.
5. Check In – After finishing, take a moment to notice any changes in tension or pain. Even subtle shifts are signs that your nervous system is responding.

This exercise helps retrain the nervous system to feel safe, reducing its need to stay on high alert. Over time, small practices like this can help rewire the brain's pain pathways, making pain less overwhelming.

The Endocannabinoid System: The Body's Built-In Pain Regulator

Lisa was beginning to understand just how deeply interconnected her body's systems were. Her nervous system had been stuck in a cycle of high alert, amplifying pain signals. Her endocrine system had been working overtime, flooding her body with stress hormones that disrupted her sleep and energy. But there was still one more system quietly shaping her experience of pain—one she had never even heard of before.

Her doctor explained it simply: "Your body has a built-in system designed to regulate pain, stress, and inflammation. It's called the endocannabinoid system, or ECS. And when it's out of balance, your entire pain experience can shift."

Lisa frowned. "Cannabinoid? Like . . . cannabis?"

Her doctor nodded. "The same receptors in your body that respond to compounds in cannabis—like CBD—are actually part of a much larger system. But your body produces its own natural cannabinoids, too, and they play a key role in managing pain."

The ECS: A Bridge Between Systems

The ECS is a vast network of receptors found throughout the brain, nervous system, immune system, and even the gut. Its main job is to maintain homeostasis—a state of balance—by regulating pain perception, inflammation, mood, and even sleep.

When functioning properly, the ECS helps to turn down the volume on pain signals and prevent inflammation from spiraling out of control. But like Lisa's other biological systems, the ECS can become dysregulated by chronic stress, pain, poor sleep, and diet.

Researchers have found that people with chronic pain often have lower levels of naturally occurring endocannabinoids, making it harder for their bodies to regulate discomfort. A 2016 study published in *Pain* suggested that endocannabinoid deficiency may be one reason some people develop conditions like fibromyalgia, migraines, and irritable bowel syndrome.

Lisa listened intently as her doctor explained how a dysfunctional ECS contributes to the pain cycle:

- Less pain modulation. When the ECS isn't functioning optimally, pain signals stay active longer than they should. This can increase pain sensitivity over time.
- Increased inflammation. The ECS helps regulate the immune system. When it's out of balance, inflammatory chemicals remain elevated, keeping pain and swelling from resolving.
- Higher stress and anxiety. Since the ECS also plays a role in emotional regulation, imbalances can lead to heightened

anxiety and stress, both of which can intensify pain perception.

"So, what do I do?" Lisa asked. "I mean, how do I get my ECS working again?"

Her doctor smiled. "Luckily, there are simple ways to support it—many of which you're already doing."

Unlike medications that work on just one system, ECS-supporting practices help regulate both pain and inflammation at the same time. These include:

- Movement. Moderate exercise, like walking, yoga, or swimming, increases the production of endocannabinoids, helping reduce pain sensitivity.
- Omega-3 fatty acids. Foods like salmon, flaxseeds, and walnuts contain compounds that help boost ECS function and regulate inflammation.
- Mindfulness and breathwork. Meditation, deep breathing, and relaxation techniques enhance endocannabinoid activity, improving stress resilience.
- Sunlight exposure. Natural light helps stimulate the production of anandamide, a key endocannabinoid often referred to as the "bliss molecule."
- CBD and other cannabinoid therapies. Some people find relief using CBD or full-spectrum hemp extracts, but these should be discussed with a healthcare provider.

Lisa realized she had already been incorporating many of these strategies into her resilience plan. But understanding how they directly influenced her ECS made her feel more empowered. She wasn't just managing symptoms—she was helping her body restore its natural ability to regulate pain.

With the nervous system and ECS in mind, Lisa was beginning to see how pain was more than just a physical sensation—it was a whole-body experience. And that meant healing needed to be whole-body, too.

THE ENDOCRINE SYSTEM: THE HIDDEN ROLE OF HORMONES IN PAIN

Lisa sat in her doctor's office, arms crossed, frustration brewing just beneath the surface. She had spent the last several months making small but meaningful changes to her routine—introducing anti-inflammatory foods, getting more movement into her day, and practicing deep breathing to calm her nervous system. And she'd been working to support her ECS. And yet, every morning, she still woke up feeling stiff and exhausted. Some days, it felt like no amount of resilience could override the deep fatigue that had settled into her bones.

Her doctor listened carefully, nodding as Lisa detailed her progress and lingering struggles. Then she said something that took Lisa by surprise.

"Your pain isn't just about your nerves or your muscles—it's about your hormones, too."

Lisa blinked. She had never considered that. Hormones? Weren't those just about emotions and metabolism? What did they have to do with pain?

Her doctor leaned forward. "The endocrine system controls so much more than we give it credit for. It regulates your energy, sleep, stress response, and even how your body processes inflammation. And when it's out of balance, it can keep the pain cycle alive."

Lisa thought back to the last few years. Her high-stress job as a realtor, the sleepless nights after her second pregnancy, the relentless exhaustion that had taken root long before her pain had even begun. It was all connected, she realized. And maybe, if she could bring her endocrine system back into balance, she could start breaking free from the cycle.

How Chronic Pain Disrupts the Endocrine System

The endocrine system is a network of glands that produce hormones—chemical messengers that help regulate nearly every function in your body. When operating smoothly, these hormones manage stress, repair tissue, regulate metabolism, and help you sleep. But chronic pain throws this finely tuned system into chaos, keeping the body in a constant state of stress and survival.

At the heart of this dysfunction is one key player: cortisol.

Cortisol is often called the "stress hormone" because it helps the body respond to immediate threats. In short bursts, it's useful—it helps you stay alert in a crisis, raises blood sugar to provide energy, and dampens pain temporarily so you can react. But in chronic pain, cortisol stops being a short-term helper and becomes a long-term disruptor.

Here's what happens when cortisol stays elevated for too long:

- Increased Inflammation: While cortisol initially reduces inflammation, prolonged exposure actually has the opposite effect. Over time, it causes immune cells to become desensitized, making inflammation worse.
- Disrupted Sleep Cycles: Normally, cortisol follows a rhythm—higher in the morning to help you wake up, lower at night to allow for deep rest. But chronic pain disrupts this cycle, leading to trouble falling and staying asleep.
- Muscle and Tissue Breakdown: High cortisol levels reduce the production of growth hormone, which is necessary for muscle repair and healing. Without it, recovery slows down, and pain persists.
- Emotional and Mental Health Challenges: Chronically high cortisol levels can contribute to anxiety, depression, and brain fog—making pain feel even more overwhelming.

Chronic Pain and Endocrine Disruption Cycle

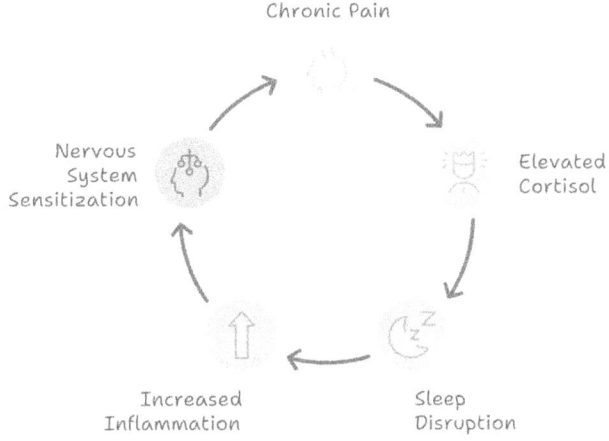

Lisa's doctor explained it simply: "Think of your body like a house. Cortisol is supposed to act like a firefighter—helping you handle occasional blazes. But with chronic pain, your body thinks there's a fire all the time. And instead of helping, the firefighter starts knocking down walls just to keep the fire at bay."

Lisa let out a breath. That was exactly how she felt—like her body was constantly bracing for impact, never able to fully rest.

The Sleep-Pain Cycle: Why Poor Sleep Makes Everything Worse

As Lisa sat with this new understanding, her doctor asked her a simple but crucial question:

"How well are you sleeping?"

Lisa almost laughed. She hadn't had a truly restful night's sleep in years. Between the pain, the stress, and the sheer exhaustion of keeping up with her family and work, her nights were restless, her mornings foggy. And no matter how much she tried to "push through" her fatigue, she always felt drained.

Her doctor nodded knowingly. "That's because chronic pain and poor sleep feed into each other. When you don't get enough deep sleep, your body doesn't produce enough growth hormone, which is essential for healing. And when you don't heal properly, your pain increases—which then makes it even harder to sleep."

This is known as the sleep-pain cycle, and it's one of the most frustrating traps for people with chronic pain:

- Pain makes it harder to sleep.
- Poor sleep reduces the body's ability to regulate stress hormones.
- Dysregulated stress hormones increase pain sensitivity.
- Increased pain makes sleep even more difficult.

That connection between sleep and hormones stuck with Lisa. Deep, restorative sleep supports not only healing but also the balance of key hormones like cortisol and melatonin. When these rhythms are disrupted, it can send the whole endocrine system out of sync—impacting everything from mood and metabolism to pain perception. In some cases, doctors may recommend short-term hormone support, like melatonin supplements or other prescriptions, to help reset the body's natural patterns. But Lisa's doctor emphasized that many people can begin restoring hormonal balance through changes to sleep habits alone.

One important factor her doctor also screened for was obstructive sleep apnea (OSA)—a condition in which breathing briefly stops during sleep, often without the person knowing. These repeated interruptions reduce oxygen levels and fragment deep sleep, worsening fatigue, inflammation, and pain sensitivity. OSA is more common than many people realize, especially in those with chronic pain. If suspected, it's vital to get assessed and treated, since unrecognized sleep apnea can make all other healing efforts less effective.

This cycle can feel impossible to escape. But Lisa's doctor reassured her: "Even small changes to your sleep routine can start to tip the balance back in your favor."

Lisa's struggles weren't unique—humans have wrestled with the impact of stress and sleep deprivation for centuries.

Before artificial lighting and the era of industrial revolution, humans naturally followed the sun's rhythm, rising with daylight and winding down at sunset. The introduction of electric light and industrial work schedules dramatically altered sleep patterns, increasing sleep deprivation.

As we are in a digital and technological revolution with changes arguably on par with those of the industrial revolution, we are again facing new challenges to sleep all the time. Today, the blue light from screens suppresses melatonin—the hormone that signals sleep—disrupting the body's natural rhythm. Studies have shown that just two hours of screen time before bed can reduce melatonin levels by 22 percent, making it harder to fall asleep.

Understanding this history helped Lisa see her struggles in a broader context—her body wasn't broken; it was responding to the same disruptions that have impacted people for generations.

Lisa left her appointment determined to take control of her sleep and hormone regulation. Instead of focusing on drastic changes, she started with small, intentional shifts that supported her body's natural rhythms, settling on a four-step plan that her doctor had helped her conceptualize.

Step 1: Creating a Consistent Sleep Routine
Lisa set a consistent bedtime and wake-up time, even on weekends. She also eliminated screens an hour before bed, switching to a book or a short meditation instead.

Step 2: Supporting Stable Blood Sugar
She had never realized how low blood sugar at night could spike cortisol, disrupting sleep. To stabilize her blood sugar, she started having a small snack before bed—a handful of almonds or a spoonful of yogurt with honey.

Step 3: Practicing a Wind-Down Ritual
Lisa introduced guided relaxation exercises to help her shift out

of stress mode before sleep. She used deep breathing, progressive muscle relaxation, and a gratitude journal to calm her nervous system.

Step 4: Adjusting Light Exposure

Lisa learned that morning sunlight exposure helped reset her cortisol rhythm. Each morning, she took her coffee outside for five minutes, letting natural light signal to her brain that it was time to be alert.

SIDEBAR

Taking Action: The 3-Day Sleep Reset Challenge

Lisa's approach to endocrine balance can work for you, too. Here's an activity to help reset your stress and sleep rhythms. For the next three days, commit to these small changes:

1. Morning Light Exposure: Spend 5-10 minutes outside within an hour of waking.
2. Blood Sugar Balance: Have a small protein-based snack before bed.
3. Screen-Free Wind-Down: Avoid screens 60 minutes before bed.
4. Breathwork for Sleep: Try a 4-7-8 breathing pattern (inhale for 4 seconds, hold for 7, exhale for 8) to calm your system.

At the end of the three days, reflect:

- Did you fall asleep faster?
- Did you wake up feeling more rested?
- Did your pain levels feel even slightly improved?

Lisa didn't notice a massive change overnight, but after a few weeks of consistency, something shifted—her mornings felt just a little lighter, her stiffness a little less severe. She came to a crucial realization: when supported right, her body wanted to rebound, to heal, to become more resilient.

And that was enough to keep going.

CHAPTER-END AFFIRMATIONS

Rebuilding Biological Balance, One System at a Time

Lisa's journey toward resilience wasn't about overpowering her pain—it was about learning how to restore balance within her body. Every system was connected, every function intertwined. Healing wasn't about pushing through; it was about learning to support the systems that sustain energy, calm pain, and foster repair.

Some days, the shifts were small—moments of deep breathing that eased the tension in her nervous system, a good night's sleep that helped regulate her hormones. Other days, progress felt invisible, but she trusted that every choice to work with her body rather than against it was part of the foundation she was rebuilding.

Biological resilience isn't about forcing healing to happen. It's about creating the conditions where healing can take root.

These affirmations are here to remind you that your body is capable of adaptation, recovery, and strength—one small choice at a time.

For My Nervous System

- My body is safe. I am not in danger, even when pain tries to convince me otherwise.
- I can help my nervous system shift out of stress mode and into a place of calm.
- Every deep breath I take reminds my body that I am in control.
- Even when my pain feels loud, I can create moments of stillness and ease.

For My Endocrine System

- I honor my body's natural rhythms and give myself the rest I need.
- Sleep is not a luxury—it is essential for my healing, my energy, and my balance.

- My hormones are not my enemy; they are part of my body's complex and beautiful design.
- I am learning to support my body's ability to restore itself, one small habit at a time.

CHAPTER-END ACTIVITY

Restoring Balance to Your Nervous and Endocrine Systems

Biological resilience is about creating the right conditions for healing—not just addressing symptoms. This activity will help you assess how your nervous system and endocrine system may be out of sync and take small, practical steps to restore balance.

Step 1: Assess Your Current Regulation
For each question, rate yourself on a scale of 1–5 (1 = needs significant improvement, 5 = feels balanced).

Nervous System (Stress & Sensory Regulation)

- Do I often feel on edge, tense, or stuck in "fight-or-flight" mode?
- Can I easily shift into a relaxed state, or does my body struggle to calm down?
- Am I using breathwork, mindfulness, or relaxation techniques to support my nervous system?

Endocrine System (Hormones & Sleep)

- Am I getting at least 7–8 hours of restorative sleep most nights?
- Do I wake up feeling refreshed, or do I often feel groggy and unwell-rested?
- Do I feel like my energy levels are steady, or do I experience frequent crashes?

Step 2: Choose One System to Focus On
Look at your scores. Which system feels most out of balance right now? Choose one to focus on this week.

- If your nervous system feels dysregulated, try a daily breathwork or progressive relaxation practice.
- If your endocrine system is struggling, improve your sleep routine, especially limiting screen time before bed.

Step 3: Track Your Progress Over Three Days

For the next three days, commit to one small, manageable action that supports the system you chose.

Each day, reflect:

- What small action did I take today to support my body?
- Did I notice even the slightest improvement in how I felt?
- What change felt the easiest or most natural to maintain?
- What's one small act of kindness I can offer my body today, even if I'm in pain?

CHAPTER 4
REBUILDING ENERGY AND REDUCING INFLAMMATION

Lisa slumped onto her couch, her body heavy with exhaustion. The pain in her back hadn't flared any more than usual today, but she still felt utterly drained. No matter how much she rested, she never seemed to feel refreshed. Even on nights when she managed to sleep, she woke up groggy, as if her body hadn't done the basic work of recharging.

She had always thought of pain as something physical—something in her muscles, nerves, or joints. But this? This was different. This was a kind of fatigue that ran deeper than tiredness, as if every cell in her body had simply run out of fuel.

At her next appointment, she voiced this frustration to her doctor.

"I just don't understand," she admitted. "I'm trying everything—breathing exercises, movement, diet. But I still feel . . . empty. Like I don't have the energy to keep going."

Her doctor nodded. "That's because chronic pain doesn't just exhaust your muscles. It drains your energy at the cellular level."

Lisa frowned. "What do you mean?"

Her doctor pulled out a diagram of a single human cell, highlighting a tiny structure inside.

"This is a mitochondrion," she explained. "It's like a battery for your body. Every cell you have is packed with these tiny powerhouses, turning food and oxygen into energy. But when you're dealing with chronic pain, these mitochondria don't function properly. They struggle to produce enough energy, and instead of fueling your body, they can actually start producing more stress and inflammation."

Lisa had never thought about energy in such a microscopic way before. She had always assumed exhaustion meant she needed more rest, more coffee, or more willpower. But what if it was her body's actual energy factories that were failing her?

THE POWERHOUSES OF THE BODY—AND WHAT HAPPENS WHEN THEY FALTER

Mitochondria are often called the powerhouses of the cell because they convert glucose, oxygen, and nutrients into ATP (adenosine triphosphate), the molecule that fuels nearly every process in the body—from muscle movement to brain function to cellular repair. When mitochondria function optimally, the body produces steady, sustained energy. But when they become dysfunctional—a process called mitochondrial dysfunction—energy production plummets, leaving people feeling constantly fatigued, mentally foggy, and physically weak.

For people with chronic pain, this dysfunction is both a cause and a consequence of their condition. Research has shown that chronic pain increases oxidative stress, a damaging process that weakens mitochondria. At the same time, low mitochondrial function means cells struggle to repair themselves, making pain worse.

A 2016 study published in *Pain Medicine* found that patients with fibromyalgia—a chronic pain condition—had significantly reduced mitochondrial function in their muscle cells. Another 2020 study in *Neuroscience & Biobehavioral Reviews* linked mitochondrial dysfunction to heightened pain sensitivity, suggesting that energy depletion plays a key role in how the body experiences chronic pain.

Lisa's doctor explained it with a simple analogy:

"Imagine trying to power a city on a failing electrical grid. The lights flicker, appliances don't work as they should, and everything is slower and less efficient. That's what happens when your mitochondria aren't producing enough energy—you feel weak, sluggish, and overwhelmed by even small tasks."

Lisa nodded slowly. "So, how do I fix my power grid?"

Her doctor smiled. "You start by giving your mitochondria what they need to thrive."

If her exhaustion was rooted in mitochondrial dysfunction, that meant there were tangible steps she could take to rebuild her energy. She made a plan focused on three core areas: nutrition, movement, and restorative habits.

She started with food. Research had shown that certain nutrients act as direct fuel for mitochondrial health, helping cells produce energy more efficiently. She made a conscious effort to include more foods rich in Coenzyme Q10, a compound found in fatty fish, nuts, and organ meats that helps mitochondria generate ATP. Magnesium was another key nutrient, essential for over 300 cellular functions, including energy conversion. She started eating more leafy greens, almonds, and dark chocolate.

Omega-3 fatty acids, found in salmon and walnuts, had anti-inflammatory properties that protected mitochondria from oxidative stress. She learned that antioxidants like vitamin C, vitamin E, and polyphenols—found in berries, green tea, and dark chocolate—could help counteract the oxidative damage that chronic pain caused at the cellular level. She even started adding a teaspoon of creatine powder to her morning smoothie, after learning that creatine helped store and transfer energy within cells.

Within two weeks, she noticed a subtle but significant shift—her body didn't feel quite as drained after daily activities, and she had more mental clarity throughout the day.

Next, she focused on movement. Lisa had always thought of exercise as something exhausting, but now she realized that the right kind of movement could actually stimulate mitochondrial growth and increase energy production. Her doctor suggested that instead of pushing herself to do long workouts, she should aim for small, frequent bursts of activity—just five minutes of movement, three times a day.

In the morning, she took a short, slow walk outside, letting the sunlight wake her up. In the afternoon, she did a few bodyweight squats and stretches to keep her muscles engaged. In the evening, she practiced five minutes of restorative yoga to help her body wind down.

This type of movement, called mitochondrial conditioning, had been studied extensively. A 2018 study in *Cell Metabolism* found that low-intensity movement, done consistently, actually increases the number of mitochondria in the body, effectively building new power plants to produce more energy.

After a month, Lisa realized she wasn't just moving more—she was recovering faster after physical activity.

Her final step was prioritizing deep rest. She'd realized the importance of sleep in supporting endocrine and immune resilience, but of course it didn't stop there. One of the biggest disruptors of mitochondrial health is poor sleep. During deep sleep, mitochondria repair themselves, cleaning out damaged cells and restoring energy levels. She committed to a strict sleep schedule, aiming for at least seven hours every night. She avoided screens before bed to prevent blue light from disrupting her melatonin production. She also had a magnesium-rich snack before bed, like almonds or yogurt, to help her muscles relax and improve sleep quality.

Within a few weeks, Lisa noticed something remarkable: she was waking up with actual energy.

SIDEBAR

Taking Action: Recharging Your Cellular Energy

If you struggle with chronic fatigue and pain, try this simple mitochondrial reset challenge:

For the next three days, commit to:

- Eating one energy-rich food per meal, such as leafy greens, fatty fish, or nuts.

- Moving gently for five minutes, three times a day, with walking, stretching, or yoga.
- Sleeping at least seven hours, with a wind-down routine to help your body transition into deep rest.

At the end of three days, reflect:

- Did you feel any increase in energy?
- Did your pain seem less overwhelming?
- Were you able to complete daily tasks with more ease?

Lisa's newfound focus on energy production helped her see her struggles in a new light. Humans evolved in environments where energy conservation was critical for survival. Anthropologists have studied how early hunter-gatherers optimized mitochondrial function through natural cycles of movement, fasting, and rest. Our ancestors ate whole, unprocessed foods rich in mitochondrial-supporting nutrients like omega-3s and antioxidants. They engaged in natural, low-intensity movement throughout the day. They prioritized restful, uninterrupted sleep because survival depended on full energy recovery.

In contrast, modern lifestyles—processed diets, sedentary habits, chronic stress—deplete mitochondrial function, making it harder for the body to sustain energy and heal from pain. Lisa realized she wasn't broken. Her body was simply responding to an energy-starved environment. And she had the power to change that.

She wasn't just enduring life anymore.

She was reclaiming her energy.

THE IMMUNE SYSTEM: QUIETING THE FIRE OF CHRONIC INFLAMMATION

Lisa sat at her kitchen table, staring at the cup of herbal tea in her hands. It was her new nighttime routine—turmeric and ginger, both anti-inflammatory, both meant to help her body heal. She wanted to believe it was making a difference, but she wasn't sure.

Lately, she had been learning about inflammation—not the kind you get from a sprained ankle or a healing cut, but the deep, hidden kind that lingers in the body for years, fueling pain from the inside out. Her doctor had explained it as a fire that never quite goes out, smoldering beneath the surface, constantly triggering pain signals.

"I don't get it," she had said at her last appointment. "I thought inflammation was supposed to be a good thing. Isn't it part of healing?"

"It is," her doctor had replied. "But only in the short term. When inflammation sticks around too long, it starts doing more harm than good."

Lisa hadn't realized it before, but her body had been trapped in a state of chronic inflammation for years—keeping her immune system on high alert, amplifying her pain, and draining her energy.

And now, she had to figure out how to calm the fire.

The immune system's job is to protect the body from harm. It fights off infections, repairs injuries, and keeps everything in balance. When you twist an ankle, for example, the immune system sends an army of white blood cells to the area, triggering swelling and heat—the classic signs of inflammation. This is a good thing. The swelling increases blood flow, delivering oxygen and nutrients to repair the damage.

But what happens when the immune system stays in this reactive state for too long?

In chronic pain conditions, inflammation doesn't resolve—it lingers. This is called chronic systemic inflammation, and it can make the nervous system hypersensitive, disrupt hormones, and worsen fatigue. Researchers have found that people with chronic pain often have elevated levels of inflammatory markers like cytokines, C-reactive protein (CRP), and interleukins—proteins that tell the immune system to stay in attack mode.

A 2019 study published in *Nature Medicine* found that chronic pain patients had immune systems that were "stuck" in a low-grade inflammatory response, making their nerves more sensitive to pain signals. Another study in *Pain* linked high inflammation levels to increased pain severity in conditions like arthritis, fibromyalgia, and even back pain.

Lisa was stunned when she learned this. She had always thought of pain as something mechanical—something wrong with her muscles, her bones, her posture. But if her immune system was actively making her pain worse, that changed everything.

The question was: how could she turn it off?

The Fire That Won't Go Out: Why Chronic Inflammation Persists

Lisa's doctor explained that several factors could keep inflammation going long after an injury had healed:

- Stress: Chronic stress causes the body to release cortisol, which in the short term suppresses inflammation, but over time, weakens the immune system's ability to regulate itself properly.
- Poor Sleep: Sleep is the body's natural reset button. Without enough deep rest, inflammatory markers like CRP and cytokines remain elevated.
- Diet: Processed foods, sugar, and unhealthy fats can contribute to "pro-inflammatory" conditions in the body, increasing oxidative stress and damaging cells.
- Environmental Toxins: Exposure to pollution, cigarette smoke, or chemicals in food and household products can keep the immune system in a constant state of activation.

Lisa realized that her life checked almost every box. She had spent years running on stress, eating whatever was easiest, and barely sleeping. No wonder her body felt like it was waging war on itself. She'd started to make strides in the last few weeks to support biological resilience, but she knew she needed to add more focused immune support into the mix.

MASTERING CHRONIC PAIN

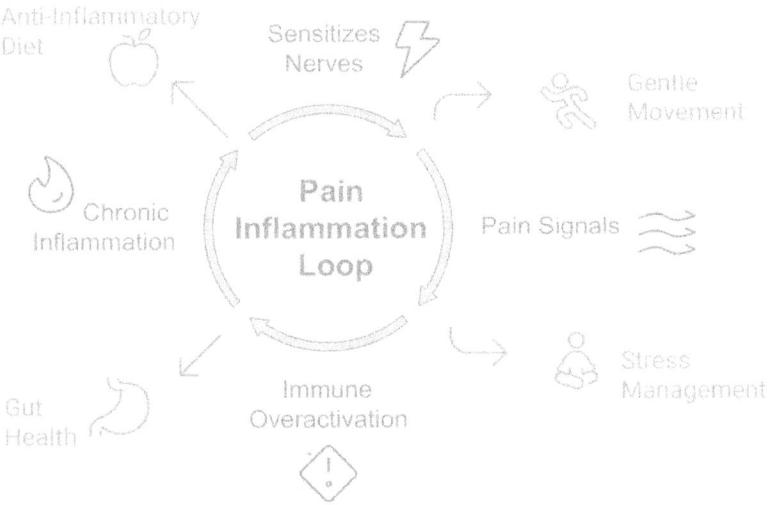

As Lisa dug deeper into the science of inflammation, she learned that it wasn't just a personal struggle—it was something deeply embedded in human history.

The immune system evolved to protect early humans from infections and wounds. In ancient times, inflammation was a life-saving response to injuries, helping hunters and gatherers recover quickly. But in modern life, we aren't facing daily survival threats. Instead, our stressors are chronic—deadlines, financial worries, social isolation. The same immune response that once saved lives is now being triggered by things that don't require a full-blown inflammatory reaction.

This shift is why so many people today struggle with chronic inflammatory diseases—arthritis, autoimmune disorders, chronic pain. Our bodies are operating on an outdated defense system, fighting battles that don't exist.

Lisa realized that her pain wasn't a sign of weakness. It was a sign that her body was still trying to protect her, even though it no longer needed to.

And that meant she had the power to reprogram it. Lisa decided to tackle inflammation from multiple angles, focusing on the things she could control.

She started with food. She had already been making small changes to support her mitochondria, but now she wanted to specifically lower inflammation. She swapped out processed snacks for anti-inflammatory foods: leafy greens, berries, turmeric, and walnuts. She cut back on sugar and refined grains. Within two weeks, she noticed she wasn't waking up as stiff in the morning.

Next, she addressed sleep. Chronic inflammation and poor sleep were a vicious cycle—the worse her sleep, the worse her inflammation, and vice versa. She set a strict bedtime, dimmed her lights in the evening, and stopped scrolling on her phone before bed. Her sleep tracker showed she was getting more deep sleep than before.

Stress was the hardest factor to change. She had never been good at slowing down, but she started using guided meditations and deep breathing exercises. Her therapist also introduced her to a concept called "vagal toning"—stimulating the Vagus nerve, which controls the body's relaxation response. She tried humming, slow breathing, and even cold-water exposure.

Over time, Lisa started noticing changes. Her pain wasn't gone, but she felt different—less reactive, less trapped in the endless loop of stress and exhaustion.

She was starting to believe that healing wasn't about fixing one thing. It was about creating an environment where her body could stop fighting itself.

SIDEBAR

Taking Action: Cooling the Inflammation Fire

If chronic inflammation is part of your pain cycle, try this three-step experiment to help reset your immune system:

1. **Choose one anti-inflammatory food to add to your meals every day for a week.** Some options include:
   - Leafy greens (spinach, kale)
   - Fatty fish (salmon, sardines)
   - Berries (blueberries, raspberries)
   - Nuts and seeds (almonds, flaxseeds)
   - Spices (turmeric, ginger)
2. **Commit to one relaxation technique for five minutes a day.** Try:
   - Diaphragmatic breathing
   - Humming or singing to stimulate the Vagus nerve
   - Progressive muscle relaxation
3. **As mentioned earlier, track your sleep for one week.** Each morning, write down:
   - How many hours you slept
   - Whether you woke up feeling rested
   - If you noticed any difference in pain levels

At the end of the week, reflect:

- Did you notice any small improvements?
- Did reducing stress or improving sleep seem to have any impact on your pain?
- What change felt easiest to maintain?

Lisa's journey with inflammation wasn't over. She was on her way to understanding what it meant to build her resilience blueprint, though. She had made huge strides in better understanding the biological systems involved in chronic pain—how her nervous system, endocrine system, mitochondrial energy system, and immune system all worked together towards balance.

She was starting to grasp the connection between body, brain, and pain more clearly and fully all the time. But there was still one major piece of the puzzle: the gut.

Her doctor had mentioned it in passing—how gut bacteria could influence pain, inflammation, even mood. At first, Lisa didn't see the connection. But as she started digging deeper, she realized that healing her pain meant healing her gut, too.

Scientists now recognize that gut bacteria don't just influence digestion—they send messages to the brain that can heighten or dampen pain. In the next chapter, we'll explore the gut-brain connection—how the trillions of microbes in your digestive system influence inflammation, stress, and even how your brain perceives pain. If calming inflammation was like putting out a fire, balancing gut health was like making sure it never sparked again.

And for Lisa, that meant her next step was clear.

She had put out the fire.

Now it was time to better understand the connection between her brain and her stomach to help keep it from coming back. Now, she needed to rebuild.

CHAPTER-END AFFIRMATIONS

Rebuilding Energy and Reducing Inflammation

Lisa wasn't just managing pain anymore—she was learning how to restore her body's energy systems and reduce chronic inflammation. Healing wasn't about pushing through exhaustion or ignoring pain signals. It was about understanding what her body needed and giving it the right kind of support.

Some days, the changes felt subtle—choosing nourishing foods that supported her immune system, moving her body in gentle, sustainable ways, prioritizing restorative sleep. Other days, it felt like nothing was working. But she reminded herself: healing isn't linear—it's a process of rebuilding strength, one step at a time.

These affirmations are here to help you trust in your body's capacity for resilience and recovery—even when progress feels slow.

For My Immune System

- I release what no longer serves me—stress, tension, and inflammation do not define me.
- Every nourishing choice I make helps my body fight less and heal more.
- My body knows how to repair itself. I trust the process of healing.
- I am not at war with my body—I am working in partnership with it.

For My Mitochondria & Energy Production

- My energy is valuable, and I choose to protect and restore it.
- Rest is not weakness—rest is rebuilding.
- Even when I feel drained, I know my body is still working for me, not against me.
- I honor my body's need for movement, nourishment, and restoration.

- I am not powerless in my healing. Every small action I take supports my body's ability to adapt, recover, and grow stronger.

CHAPTER-END ACTIVITY

Rebuilding Energy and Reducing Inflammation

Now that you've explored how stress and sleep impact pain, it's time to restore energy production and lower inflammation. This activity will help you assess how your immune system and mitochondria may be contributing to your symptoms and take targeted action.

Step 1: Assess Your Energy and Inflammation Levels

For each question, rate yourself on a scale of 1–5 (1 = needs significant improvement, 5 = feels balanced).

Immune System (Inflammation & Recovery)

- Do I often feel inflamed (stiff joints, bloating, chronic swelling, or recurring illness)?
- Have I been mindful of anti-inflammatory nutrition, stress management, and sleep?
- Am I giving my body enough time and support to repair itself?

Mitochondria & Energy Production (Cellular Resilience)

- Do I often feel deep fatigue, even when I've rested?
- Am I fueling my body with nutrient-rich, energy-supporting foods?
- Have I been incorporating gentle movement into my routine to stimulate energy production?

Step 2: Choose One System to Focus On

Look at your scores. Which system feels most out of balance right now? Choose one to focus on this week.

If your immune system feels overactive, add one anti-inflammatory food per meal and track how you feel.

If your energy production feels depleted, commit to three short movement breaks per day to gently recharge your mitochondria.

Step 3: Track Your Progress Over Three Days

For the next three days, commit to one small, manageable action that supports the system you chose.

Each day, reflect:

- What small action did I take today to support my body?
- Did I notice even the slightest improvement in how I felt?
- What change felt the easiest or most natural to maintain?
- What's one thing I can do today to help my body recover energy gently and naturally?

CHAPTER 5

THE GUT-BRAIN CONNECTION: A CONVERSATION BETWEEN BODY AND MIND

When her doctor had first mentioned the gut-brain connection, Lisa was uncertain.

But desperation has a way of softening resistance. She wasn't ready to believe food could change her pain, but she was willing to try. She started small: a handful of spinach tossed into her eggs, a glass of water in place of soda. These weren't drastic changes, just tiny experiments—an offering to her body, though she wasn't sure if it would notice.

After just a few weeks, Lisa was seeing a difference.

She realized she wasn't waking up quite as stiff. The fog of exhaustion that had clung to her mornings for years felt lighter. When she ate the pastries she once devoured without a second thought, she felt sluggish, like her body was rejecting them outright. She had never noticed these patterns before. But now, she was paying attention.

Curious, she began to read about the gut-brain connection, about how the trillions of bacteria in her gut weren't just digesting food but communicating with her nervous system, influencing inflammation, even shaping how she processed pain. It wasn't just about digestion—it was about resilience, about how her body responded to the world around it.

She took another small step. A probiotic yogurt at breakfast. A handful of almonds in place of a granola bar. It didn't feel like she was overhauling her life, just nudging it in a different direction. But little by little, the changes began to add up. Her pain wasn't gone, but it was less sharp, less consuming. Her energy no longer abandoned her by midafternoon. And perhaps most importantly, she began to feel something she hadn't felt in years—a sense of control.

There were still hard days, still moments when the pain pushed back. But for the first time, she wasn't waiting to be saved. She was part of her own healing.

SIDEBAR

Take Action: Add One Gut-Friendly Habit to Your Routine

The gut-brain axis acts as a two-way communication system between your gut and brain, influencing your mood, stress response, and pain levels. When this connection is disrupted by poor diet or stress, it can amplify chronic pain.

- Include a serving of probiotic food like yogurt or sauerkraut.
- Drink a glass of water with each meal to support digestion.
- Take two minutes to breathe deeply, calming your gut-brain connection.

HOW YOUR GUT DRIVES CHRONIC PAIN

Your gut does far more than digest food—it is a command center that communicates directly with your brain, influencing everything from mood to inflammation to how intensely you experience pain. This connection, known as the gut-brain axis, is a sophisticated network linking the digestive system with the nervous system. When this relationship is functioning well, it helps regulate pain, manage stress, and support overall resilience. But when gut health is disrupted, it can tip the body into a cycle of heightened pain sensitivity and chronic inflammation.

At the heart of this connection is the enteric nervous system, a vast web of nerves embedded in the gut. This system functions semi-independently but stays in constant dialogue with the brain through the Vagus nerve—one of the body's main communication highways. The Vagus nerve regulates stress responses, inflammation, and pain perception. When gut health is stable, the signals moving along this pathway help maintain balance. But when gut function is impaired—due to poor diet, chronic stress, or inflammation—these signals shift from regulating resilience to reinforcing distress, increasing the nervous system's sensitivity to pain.

Gut-Brain Communication via Vagus Nerve

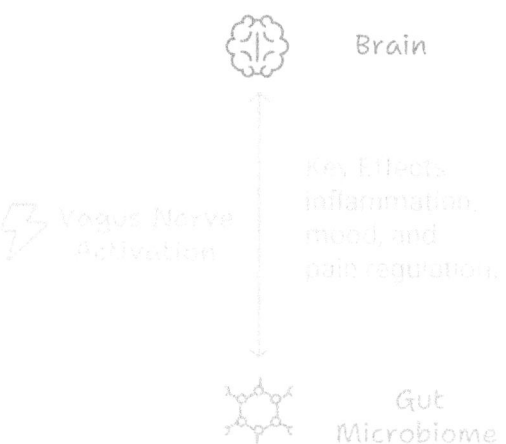

Beyond its role in nerve signaling, the gut also serves as a biochemical powerhouse, producing nearly 90% of the body's serotonin—the neurotransmitter that stabilizes mood and plays a crucial role in how the brain perceives pain. This is why the gut is often referred to as the second brain. When its balance is disrupted, serotonin production drops, leaving the nervous system more vulnerable to stress and pain, while emotional resilience declines.

The gut's influence extends even further through the gut microbiome—the trillions of bacteria, fungi, and microbes that reside in the digestive tract. These microbes regulate immune responses, help manage inflammation and even produce molecules that shape brain function. Some researchers estimate that up to 30% of the molecules in your bloodstream originate from gut microbes, affecting everything from stress resilience to immune regulation. When the microbiome is thriving, these molecules promote healing and stability. But when it is out of balance, inflammation increases, stress compounds, and the nervous system remains in a reactive state—fueling chronic pain.

A damaged gut lining can also contribute to this cycle. In a healthy gut, the intestinal lining acts as a barrier, allowing only beneficial nutrients into the bloodstream. But when this barrier is compromised—a condition often called leaky gut syndrome—toxins, undigested food particles, and harmful microbes escape, triggering an immune response. The body, sensing a threat, releases inflammatory chemicals that spread beyond the gut, amplifying pain signals in the nervous system and making pain feel more intense and persistent.

The effects of gut dysfunction aren't just physical. Disruptions in gut health can fuel emotional distress, making it harder to cope with stress and more difficult to manage pain. When serotonin production in the gut falters, resilience weakens, and feelings of anxiety or depression can intensify. This further reinforces pain pathways, trapping the body in a self-perpetuating loop of discomfort and stress.

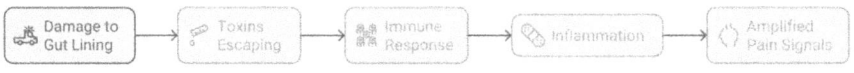

The good news is that healing the gut can help break this cycle. A well-functioning gut doesn't just support digestion—it acts as a stabilizer, buffering against life's stresses and regulating pain. By nurturing the gut through targeted nutrition, stress management, and lifestyle changes, you can calm an overactive nervous system, reduce inflammation, and restore balance to the entire body.

The Peak Resilience Method takes this holistic approach, recognizing that a strong, balanced gut supports not just digestion, but the entire web of systems that govern healing, adaptability, and long-term resilience. When your gut is in harmony, pain signals quiet down, stress responses soften, and your body regains its ability to heal.

SIDEBAR

Take Action: Vagus Nerve Activation Practice

Sit comfortably and take five slow, deep breaths, expanding your belly as you inhale and letting it fall naturally as you exhale. This simple practice stimulates the Vagus nerve, enhancing communication between your gut and brain.

> **Journal Prompt:** *After practicing Vagus nerve activation, write down any changes in how your body or mind feels. Did you notice a sense of calm or reduced tension?*

THE GUT'S ROLE IN INTERNAL SYSTEM SABOTAGE

In earlier chapters, we explored how chronic pain disrupts the body's internal systems—keeping the nervous system on high alert, flooding the body with stress hormones, and triggering immune overreactions that sustain inflammation. These disruptions create a state of internal system sabotage, where the body gets trapped in cycles of pain, stress, and dysfunction.

But what if there were a way to interrupt this cycle at the source? Increasingly, research is pointing to the gut as one of the most powerful regulators of these internal systems. Far from being just a digestive organ, the gut is a control center—sending signals that can either calm or amplify pain, regulate or disrupt hormones, and balance or inflame the immune response.

This connection is largely governed by the gut microbiome, the trillions of bacteria, fungi, and other microbes living in the digestive tract. These microbes interact with nearly every major system in the body, shaping everything from mood to metabolism to how the brain perceives pain. When the microbiome is thriving, it supports balance across these systems. But when gut health is compromised—through poor diet, chronic stress, or other factors—it can worsen pain, weaken stress resilience, and fuel inflammation.

Let's take a closer look at how gut health influences the nervous, endocrine, and immune systems—and how supporting the gut can help restore balance where pain has taken over.

The Gut-Nervous System Connection

Earlier, we explored how an overactive nervous system can intensify pain by keeping the body in a constant state of fight-or-flight. The gut plays a key role in regulating this response. Through the Vagus nerve, the gut sends signals that can either calm the nervous system—lowering pain sensitivity—or keep it on high alert.

An inflamed gut, or one with an imbalanced microbiome, can send distress signals to the brain, reinforcing the fight-or-flight state and increasing pain sensitivity. On the other hand, a well-supported gut can help tone down these pain signals, creating a more stable nervous system that doesn't react as intensely to stress or discomfort.

The Gut-Endocrine System Connection

The endocrine system, which regulates hormones like cortisol (stress hormone) and serotonin (mood and pain regulator), is deeply influenced by the gut. Chronic pain often keeps cortisol levels elevated, which can disrupt sleep, weaken the immune system, and make pain feel worse.

The gut helps regulate this process in two ways:

Microbiome balance – A healthy gut microbiome helps maintain steady cortisol levels, preventing the prolonged stress response that contributes to chronic pain.

Neurotransmitter production – As noted earlier, up to 90% of the body's serotonin is produced in the gut. When gut health is compromised, serotonin production drops, which can increase pain sensitivity, heighten stress, and weaken emotional resilience.

The Gut-Immune System Connection

The immune system relies on the gut to regulate inflammation—a key driver of chronic pain. A healthy gut microbiome produces compounds that keep inflammation in check, preventing the immune system from overreacting.

However, when the gut barrier is compromised—a condition often referred to as leaky gut—harmful substances escape into the bloodstream, triggering widespread inflammation. This chronic immune activation doesn't just affect digestion; it amplifies pain signals throughout the body.

As Lisa started to focus on gut health—integrating fiber-rich foods, probiotics, and anti-inflammatory choices—Lisa began to notice shifts. Her nervous system felt less reactive, her sleep improved, and her body seemed less locked in a state of tension. She wasn't just managing symptoms anymore—she was addressing the underlying disruptions that had been keeping her pain alive.

This is why improving gut health is a crucial step toward resilience.

By calming inflammation, rebalancing the microbiome, and supporting healthy hormone levels, the gut helps restore harmony among the nervous, endocrine, and immune systems. Strengthening the gut doesn't just reduce pain; it creates the conditions for real healing, allowing the body to move from survival mode into a state of long-term recovery.

For Lisa, this realization was empowering. Every small step she took—every nourishing meal, every moment of stress relief—wasn't just about her gut. It was about reclaiming control over her entire system.

The Peak Resilience Method emphasizes these small, strategic steps. Whether it's incorporating probiotics, managing stress, or improving diet, these changes disrupt the feedback loops that sustain chronic pain. By focusing on the gut, you're not just improving digestion—you're creating a ripple effect that restores balance across your entire body.

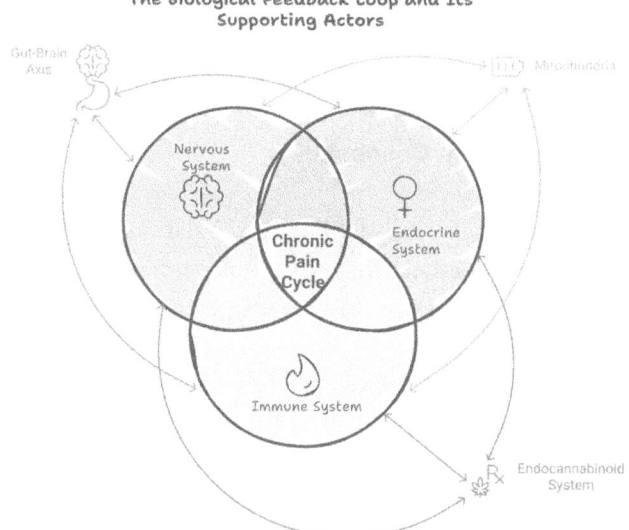

STRESS AS A CATALYST FOR GUT DYSFUNCTION

Lisa was starting to grasp how much the stress-gut connection was keeping her in a loop of pain. It wasn't just the food she ate—it was the daily pressures, the tension she carried in her gut. When she started breathing exercises before meals, she wasn't expecting much. But within days, her bloating eased, and she felt less wired before bed.

She wasn't imagining it. Her doctor explained that stress and gut health are deeply intertwined, and that Lisa was caught in a loop where pain, stress, and gut dysfunction were feeding off each other.

When the body encounters stress—whether from a difficult day, emotional strain, or even the ongoing burden of chronic pain—it activates the fight-or-flight response. The brain releases cortisol and adrenaline to help the body react to a perceived threat. But these stress hormones also divert resources away from digestion, slowing gut motility and reducing blood flow to the intestines. Over time, this suppression can disrupt the microbiome, weakening its ability to regulate inflammation, absorb nutrients, and support neurotransmitter production.

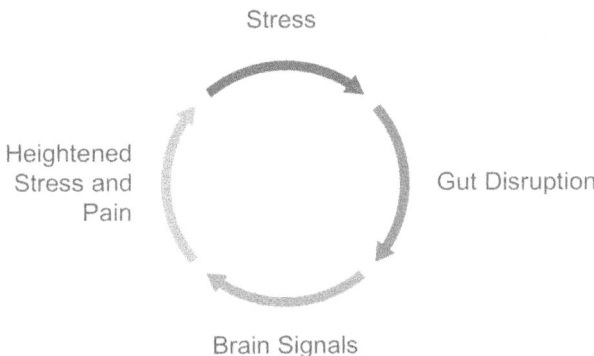

This cycle was keeping Lisa stuck. When her stress levels spiked, her digestion worsened, her pain intensified, and sleep became elusive. And the worse she slept, the more reactive her nervous system became, making the next day even harder. It was a feedback loop, reinforcing her body's internal system sabotage.

But breaking the cycle was possible. Lisa's first step was small but intentional—spending five minutes each morning practicing deep breathing before she started her day. She also experimented with small dietary changes, like incorporating fiber-rich foods and fermented options to support her gut. Within a few weeks, she began to notice subtle shifts. The worst of her bloating subsided, and her pain felt less consuming on days when she was able to keep her stress in check.

Stress may be unavoidable, but its impact on the body isn't inevitable. By learning to regulate the stress response—through mindfulness, breathwork, and gut-supportive nutrition—Lisa found she could help her body recover instead of getting stuck in survival mode.

SIDEBAR

Take Action: Mindfulness Moment

Set aside two minutes to close your eyes and focus on your breathing. As you inhale, think of a word like "calm." As you exhale, imagine releasing stress. This small practice can counteract the stress response that disrupts your gut.

Now think about how you currently respond to stress.

Could a simple practice, like mindful breathing, help break the cycle of stress and gut disruption?

BUILDING RESILIENCE THROUGH GUT HEALTH

Centuries ago, traditional medicine systems like Ayurveda and Chinese medicine understood that digestion played a key role in overall health. Modern research has confirmed what these early healers intuitively knew. Breakthrough studies on the gut microbiome have shown that these trillions of bacteria influence not just digestion—they help regulate mood, immune function, and inflammation, all of which shape how pain is experienced.

Lisa saw this firsthand as she slowly shifted her diet. She hadn't expected much from eating more fiber, cutting back on sugar, or adding probiotic-rich foods like yogurt and kimchi to her meals. But within weeks, something shifted. Her morning stiffness wasn't as severe. She had more energy throughout the day. The foods she had once eaten without thought—processed snacks, heavy meals—now left her feeling sluggish and inflamed. She began paying attention, noting patterns, and realizing just how much her gut was influencing her body's ability to recover.

The gut is a key player in resilience, shaping the body's ability to calm overactive pain signals, manage inflammation, and restore balance across multiple systems. Certain foods can help nurture this balance. Probiotics replenish beneficial bacteria, while prebiotic-rich foods like garlic, onions, and asparagus help those bacteria thrive. Hydration also plays a critical role, ensuring the gut lining stays strong and reducing the likelihood of leaky gut—a condition where toxins escape into the bloodstream, triggering widespread inflammation.

Beyond food, Lisa also learned that her stress levels were impacting her gut. Modern research has confirmed that the gut-brain axis is a two-way street. Chronic stress alters gut bacteria, increasing inflammation and reducing serotonin production—one reason why stress and pain so often go hand in hand. But the opposite is also true: by managing stress, the gut can recover. Lisa started using deep breathing exercises before meals, taking slow walks after dinner, and prioritizing small moments of calm. She didn't need to overhaul her life; even minor changes made a difference.

Tracking these shifts became part of her healing. A simple journal helped her connect certain foods to pain flare-ups, revealing hidden sensitivities. Many people, she learned, react to common triggers—not always immediately, but sometimes hours or days later.

UNCOVERING FOOD INTOLERANCES AND HIDDEN TRIGGERS

As Lisa continued refining her diet, she became aware of how some foods, even those labeled as "healthy," didn't sit well with her body. She learned that for many people, food sensitivities can create inflammation, disrupt gut bacteria, and heighten pain.

Certain ingredients are common culprits. Gluten, found in wheat, barley, and rye, can be particularly problematic for individuals with sensitivity or intolerance, as it weakens the gut lining and contributes to leaky gut syndrome. Seed oils, widely used in processed foods, contain high levels of omega-6 fatty acids, which can drive inflammation when consumed in excess. Sugar, too, can be a major disruptor, feeding harmful gut bacteria and fueling imbalances that worsen both pain and stress.

The tricky part was that Lisa didn't always react immediately to these foods. She might eat something one day and not notice an increase in pain or fatigue until the next. This delayed response made it difficult to pinpoint triggers without careful observation. Through tracking her meals and symptoms, she began recognizing patterns—certain foods left her more bloated, more fatigued, or more prone to pain flare-ups.

Not everyone reacts to the same foods, and not all intolerances look the same. Some people struggle with high-fiber foods like beans or cruciferous vegetables, while others might find dairy or nightshades problematic. Lisa experimented with an elimination diet, temporarily removing common triggers and reintroducing them one at a time. This helped her identify which foods supported her resilience and which worked against it.

The goal wasn't to restrict or fear food—it was to make informed choices. The more Lisa understood what worked for her, the more empowered she felt. Gut health wasn't just about what she added to her diet; it was also about knowing what to avoid.

SIDEBAR

Tack Action: Tools to Use

Elimination Diet Starter Plan

For two weeks, try cutting out common triggers like gluten, seed oils, or sugar. Reintroduce one at a time to see how your body responds.

Symptom Journal Prompt

Log physical and emotional symptoms as you experiment with your diet. Pay attention to delayed reactions.

Quick-Start Guide: One-Day Anti-Inflammatory Meal Plan

- Breakfast: Spinach and mushroom omelet with a side of blueberries.
- Lunch: Quinoa salad with grilled salmon, arugula, cherry tomatoes, and olive oil dressing.
- Dinner: Baked chicken breast with roasted sweet potatoes, steamed broccoli, and a sprinkle of walnuts.
- Snacks: A handful of almonds or a small serving of Greek yogurt with flaxseeds.
- Hydration Tip: Drink water infused with lemon or cucumber throughout the day to stay hydrated.

MOVING FORWARD WITH AWARENESS AND BALANCE

Lisa's journey wasn't about perfection. It was about learning to listen to her body in a new way. Scientists now know that gut health is deeply personal—what works for one person may not work for another. Lisa's path forward wasn't about following rigid rules, but about making small, thoughtful choices that supported her gut, her nervous system, and ultimately, her resilience.

Each change she made—choosing a gut-friendly meal, pausing for a deep breath, moving her body—was a quiet act of reclaiming her life from pain. The gut-brain connection, once an abstract concept, had become a tangible force in her healing.

And it wasn't just her digestion that was improving. It was her entire sense of well-being.

Lisa had spent so much of her journey focused on the physical—her back pain, her diet, her inflammation—that she hadn't considered how deeply her thoughts, emotions, and past experiences were shaping her pain. But as she began noticing patterns, she saw how stress, fear, and even memories of pain could intensify what she felt in her body.

Her gut health had given her a foundation for resilience, but it was only part of the picture. Pain isn't just physical; it is also shaped by the nervous system's response to stress, past trauma, and even unconscious habits of thought. The brain and body are constantly in conversation, and just as gut health can influence pain, so too can the mind's interpretation of it.

In Part Two, we move beyond biology to explore the psychological systems that sustain chronic pain—and, more importantly, the strategies that help rewire them. Psychological resilience isn't about ignoring pain or forcing positivity; it's about understanding how pain is processed in the brain and learning to shift those patterns. It's about retraining the nervous system, reshaping thought loops that reinforce suffering, and building a new relationship with discomfort. In the next chapter, we'll begin this process by exploring how the brain perceives pain, why past experiences influence the present, and how simple cognitive and emotional shifts can start breaking pain's hold. The work you've done to support your body is now the foundation for the next step: strengthening your mind's role in resilience.

CHAPTER-END RESOURCE

Your Guided Gut-Brain Plan for Resilience

Small, consistent actions can have a profound impact on your gut health, pain levels, and overall resilience. Use this guided plan to support your gut-brain connection and track your progress along the way.

Step 1: Nourish Your Microbiome
   Support a balanced gut ecosystem with intentional food choices:

- Probiotics: Add a daily serving of yogurt, kefir, or fermented vegetables like sauerkraut or kimchi.
- Prebiotics: Incorporate fiber-rich foods such as garlic, onions, bananas, or asparagus to feed beneficial gut bacteria.
- Reduce Disruptors: Limit processed foods, excess sugar, and seed oils, which can contribute to gut inflammation and imbalance.

Step 2: Hydrate for Gut Health
   Water plays a vital role in digestion and gut lining integrity. Aim for at least eight glasses a day, adjusting for your body's needs. Pairing hydration with fiber-rich foods—like oats, beans, or leafy greens—can further enhance digestion and gut resilience.

Step 3: Manage Stress to Support Digestion
   Chronic stress weakens gut function, but simple practices can help regulate the gut-brain connection:

- Try Mindfulness: Set aside five minutes for quiet reflection or deep breathing.
- Activate the Vagus Nerve: Use diaphragmatic breathing (slow, deep belly breaths) to stimulate relaxation.

- Practice Gratitude: End your day by listing three things you're grateful for—this small shift can reduce stress hormones and improve gut function.

Step 4: Move with Purpose

Gentle movement supports digestion and reduces inflammation:

- Take a 15-minute walk after meals to aid digestion.
- Try yoga or tai chi to combine movement with stress relief.
- Prioritize consistency: Even small, daily movements can strengthen the gut-brain connection.

Step 5: Track Your Progress

Keeping a journal can help identify what's supporting your gut health and what may be causing setbacks. Use the table below to log your meals, mood, and pain levels:

Date	Food/Drink	Mood	Pain Level (1-10)	Delayed Reactions

Reflection Questions

- Did you notice any changes in how your body responded to different foods?
- Were there any stressors that seemed to trigger digestive discomfort or pain?
- What small shift felt easiest to maintain?

By making these small adjustments, you're not just improving gut health—you're creating a foundation for resilience across your entire body. Each step brings you closer to a stronger, healthier you. What's one change you can commit to today?

CHAPTER-END ACTIVITY

Strengthening Your Gut-Brain Awareness

Gut health plays a vital role in regulating pain, mood, and overall resilience. By making small, intentional changes and tracking your body's responses, you can begin to identify patterns that may be keeping you stuck in cycles of pain and inflammation. This activity is designed to help you tune into the connection between what you eat, how you feel, and how your body responds.

Step 1: Start a Food-Mood-Pain Journal

For the next week, track the following after each meal:

- What you ate – Be as specific as possible, including ingredients and portion sizes.
- How you felt emotionally – Note any shifts in mood, energy levels, or mental clarity.
- Pain levels – Use a scale of 1 to 10, with 1 being no pain and 10 being severe pain.
- Any delayed reactions – Pay attention to symptoms that show up hours or even a day later, such as bloating, fatigue, joint stiffness, or brain fog.

This journal will help you uncover potential gut-health triggers—such as sugar, gluten, or processed foods—and recognize how dietary choices influence your pain and well-being.

Step 2: Identify Patterns

At the end of the week, review your journal. Ask yourself:

- Do certain foods or food groups seem to increase my pain or fatigue?

- Are there meals that leave me feeling more energized and balanced?
- Do I notice delayed symptoms after eating processed or inflammatory foods?
- How does my stress level affect my digestion and pain?

Step 3: Make One Small Change

Choose one simple change to support your gut health. This might include:

- Reducing processed foods or refined sugar
- Adding more fiber-rich, prebiotic foods (garlic, onions, asparagus, bananas)
- Incorporating fermented foods (yogurt, kimchi, sauerkraut)
- Drinking more water to support digestion
- Practicing deep breathing before meals to activate the Vagus nerve and aid digestion

Commit to this change for the next few days and continue tracking how you feel. Small adjustments can create a ripple effect, helping you take back control of your gut health and, in turn, your pain resilience.

> **Reflection Prompt**: *What foods or habits do you suspect might be contributing to your pain? How has tracking your meals and symptoms helped you recognize patterns? What is one thing you can do today to support your gut-brain connection?*

By taking these small, mindful steps, you're not just improving your digestion—you're strengthening the foundation for resilience, healing, and long-term well-being.

PART THREE:
PSYCHOLOGICAL RESILIENCE – REWIRING THE MIND

CHAPTER 6
PSYCHOLOGICAL SYSTEMS IN CHRONIC PAIN

Like many people we've seen over the years, met in this book, and perhaps like you, Andre used to think of his pain as a permanent feature of his life—a shadow that followed him everywhere, no matter what he did. After years of back pain from an old soccer injury, he had tried everything: physical therapy, medications, even surgery. The pain always came back. No matter how much effort he put in, it felt like his body had turned against him.

He noticed it most on days when the pain flared unexpectedly. His thoughts spiraled: *Why can't I control this? Why does my body hate me?* The frustration wasn't just a passing reaction; it stuck with him, deepening his exhaustion. And the worse he felt emotionally, the worse his pain became. It was as though his emotions and physical pain were feeding off each other in an endless loop.

His breakthrough didn't come from another medication or procedure—it came from a conversation. A friend, seeing his frustration, suggested he talk to a pain psychologist. At first, Andre bristled at the idea. "I don't need therapy," he thought. "I need my body to stop hurting." But with nothing to lose, he agreed to one session.

The psychologist explained something Andre had never considered: his brain had created well-worn pathways linking pain with fear, frustration, and helplessness. Over time, these pathways had strengthened, making his pain feel more consuming. But just as his brain had learned these patterns, it could also learn new ones.

Skeptical but intrigued, Andre tried an exercise his psychologist suggested. The next time his pain spiked, he paused. Instead of reacting with frustration, he took a slow breath and told himself: *This is a moment of discomfort, but I don't have to fight it.* It felt unnatural at first, like trying to steer a ship with an invisible wheel. But after a few weeks, he noticed a small shift. His pain wasn't gone, but he didn't feel as emotionally hijacked by it.

He started to call his pain *background noise* instead of a *constant battle*. The difference was subtle but profound—he was no longer bracing against every sensation. Slowly, he began integrating other techniques: breathing exercises, brief meditations, even just noticing when his thoughts fueled his pain. It wasn't about ignoring his body; it was about retraining his nervous system to stop overreacting. And for the first time in years, he began to believe that change was possible.

HOW CHRONIC PAIN CHANGES THE BRAIN

Andre always assumed his pain was a mechanical problem—something in his back that was injured, something physical that needed to be fixed. But after years of searching for solutions, he began to realize the pain wasn't just in his body; it was in his thoughts, his emotions, and his reactions to everyday stress.

Have you ever noticed that when you feel worse emotionally, you feel worse physically? Andre would have a particularly bad flare-up, and before he knew it, his mind was spiraling back to the same story: *Why can't I control this? Why does my body hate me?* The worse he felt emotionally, the worse his pain seemed to become. It wasn't until he started working with a pain psychologist that he learned why.

Chronic pain rewires the brain itself. Your brain is designed to adapt based on experience, a process called neuroplasticity. In many ways, neuroplasticity is what allows us to learn, grow, and recover from injury. But when pain becomes chronic, this same ability can work against you.

Repeated pain signals strengthen pathways in the brain, making it more sensitive to pain and harder to turn those signals off.

Historically, pain was thought to be a one-way street: tissue damage triggered pain, and once the injury healed, the pain stopped. But in the 1960s, researchers Ronald Melzack and Patrick Wall introduced the Gate Control Theory of Pain, which proposed that the nervous system plays an active role in shaping pain signals before they even reach the brain. Their work laid the foundation for modern pain science, showing that pain is not just a reflection of injury—it's also deeply influenced by the brain itself.

Fast forward to today, and brain imaging studies have confirmed just how much chronic pain alters the nervous system. Research shows that people with long-term pain process pain differently from those without it. In a healthy brain, pain activates areas responsible for physical sensations, like the sensory cortex. But in people with chronic pain, those signals spread to parts of the brain that regulate emotions, memories, and even self-identity. This helps explain why chronic pain often feels overwhelming: it's not just physical, it also affects emotions, thoughts, and mental well-being.

As one session with the pain psychologist quickly became many, Andre began to understand how several key areas of the brain undergo changes with chronic pain.

The Amygdala: The Brain's Alarm System

The amygdala is often described as the brain's "fear center," responsible for detecting threats and initiating the fight-or-flight response. This small, almond-shaped structure deep in the brain evolved to keep us safe from immediate danger, such as predators or other survival threats. However, in chronic pain, the amygdala becomes overactive, treating pain itself as a constant threat.

Research has shown that in individuals with chronic pain, the amygdala remains highly engaged, even in the absence of acute injury. A 2019 study in the journal *PAIN* found that people with chronic lower back pain exhibited heightened amygdala activity, leading to increased pain perception and emotional distress. This overactivation keeps the nervous system on high alert, making the body hypersensitive to pain signals.

Additionally, the amygdala is deeply connected to memory and emotion, meaning that past experiences of pain or trauma can reinforce its overactivity. This is why chronic pain sufferers often feel heightened anxiety and stress, as the amygdala continuously signals a state of perceived danger. Practices like mindfulness and meditation have been shown to reduce amygdala activation, helping to retrain the brain's response to pain stimuli.

The Prefrontal Cortex: The Brain's Regulator

The prefrontal cortex (PFC) sits at the front of the brain and plays a critical role in rational thinking, emotional regulation, and decision-making. It acts as the brain's executive center, helping to regulate impulses, manage stress, and shift focus from negative thoughts. However, in chronic pain, this region becomes compromised, weakening the ability to regulate pain-related distress.

A 2013 study published in *The Journal of Neuroscience* found that individuals with chronic pain exhibited reduced gray matter volume in the PFC, particularly in areas responsible for emotional control. This atrophy can make it harder to manage stress, reframe negative thoughts, or engage in behaviors that promote healing.

Historically, pain research focused primarily on sensory pathways, but studies in the last two decades have highlighted the PFC's essential role in pain modulation. Interestingly, therapies such as cognitive behavioral therapy (CBT) and mindfulness meditation have been shown to increase PFC activity, strengthening emotional regulation and pain resilience. By retraining the PFC, individuals can develop a greater sense of control over their pain experience.

The Sensory Cortex: Where Pain Feels Louder

The sensory cortex, or somatosensory cortex, processes physical sensations, mapping pain, touch, temperature, and body awareness. This region is crucial for distinguishing between different types of sensory input and localizing pain. However, in chronic pain, the sensory cortex undergoes changes that heighten pain perception.

A landmark 2008 study in *The Journal of Pain* used fMRI scans to show that people with fibromyalgia (a chronic pain condition) had significantly larger sensory cortex activation than healthy controls when exposed to the same pain stimulus. This suggests that the brain of a chronic pain sufferer is physically amplifying pain signals.

Another striking finding is that people with phantom limb pain—pain felt in a limb that has been amputated—show abnormal activity in the sensory cortex, demonstrating that pain perception is not solely tied to physical injury but rather how the brain interprets and processes sensory information.

These findings support the idea that neuroplasticity-based interventions, such as visualization, graded motor imagery, and mirror therapy, can help rewire the sensory cortex and reduce pain intensity. By engaging the brain in new ways, individuals can reshape how pain is processed and perceived.

The Default Mode Network (DMN): The Loop of Negative Thoughts

The default mode network (DMN) is a set of interconnected brain regions that become active when the mind is at rest—when we're daydreaming, reflecting, or thinking about ourselves. While essential for processing memories and emotions, in chronic pain sufferers, the DMN can become stuck in loops of rumination, catastrophizing, and self-referential thinking—all of which worsen pain perception.

Robert Wright's *Why Buddhism Is True* discusses how meditation helps break the DMN's grip, preventing the mind from getting caught in repetitive, distressing thought patterns. Similarly, research in neuroscience has found that people with chronic pain have hyperactive DMN activity, which correlates with greater pain severity and emotional suffering.

A 2015 study in *The Journal of Neuroscience* found that individuals with chronic pain showed increased DMN connectivity with the amygdala and sensory cortex, reinforcing both emotional distress and heightened pain perception. This explains why many chronic pain sufferers feel like their pain dominates their identity—because their brain is continuously looping through pain-related thoughts.

The good news?

Neuroplasticity works *both ways*.

Just as chronic pain strengthens unhelpful pathways, the brain is also capable of building new ones. Studies have shown that mindfulness practices can calm the amygdala, gratitude exercises can strengthen the prefrontal cortex, and visualization techniques can reshape how the sensory cortex interprets pain. With the right tools, these neural pathways can be rewired to reduce suffering and improve resilience.

For Andre, understanding that his brain wasn't "broken" but simply conditioned by years of chronic pain was a turning point. If his pain could shape his brain, then maybe his thoughts, emotions, and actions could reshape it in return. It wasn't about ignoring the pain—it was about teaching his brain to process it differently.

Your brain is adaptable. Even if chronic pain has rewired it in ways that make life harder, you can create new neural pathways that lead to relief, resilience, and hope for a better future.

SIDEBAR

Take Action: What's Your Pattern?

How do you typically react to pain emotionally? What thoughts or feelings come up when you're in pain?

Can you think of a time when a small mental shift—like focusing on gratitude—helped you feel better emotionally or physically? How could you apply that to your pain experience?

WHY PSYCHOLOGICAL TOOLS HAVE BEEN OVERLOOKED

For decades, the medical model of pain focused almost exclusively on the body. If something hurt, it must be because of tissue damage, inflammation, or a mechanical dysfunction. While these factors are important, the role of the brain and nervous system was often dismissed.

As a result, psychological tools for pain were seen with skepticism—by both patients and doctors. Some believed that addressing thoughts and emotions meant the pain wasn't *real* (which couldn't be further from the truth). Others worried that focusing on the brain implied a lack of solutions for the body. But over the last two decades, neuroscience has transformed how we understand pain.

Studies using brain imaging have shown that chronic pain rewires the brain, strengthening pathways that amplify discomfort even when the original injury has healed. Researchers have also found that mindfulness-based interventions—once dismissed as "soft" approaches—can physically alter brain activity, reducing pain-related activation in areas like the amygdala and prefrontal cortex.

One landmark study from 2016, published in *JAMA Internal Medicine*, found that mindfulness-based stress reduction (MBSR) was more effective at reducing chronic low back pain than standard medical care. Another study from the National Institutes of Health showed that cognitive behavioral therapy (CBT) could significantly reduce pain intensity and improve daily function—sometimes more effectively than opioids.

This shift isn't just happening in research labs—it's reshaping mainstream medicine. Many hospitals now integrate pain psychology, and elite athletes, military personnel, and high-performing professionals increasingly use these methods to build resilience. What was once seen as *alternative* is now *essential*. Science has confirmed what ancient healing traditions understood for centuries: the mind and body are not separate. Treating pain effectively means addressing both.

Despite this growing body of research, many people still hesitate to explore psychological approaches to pain. Some feel intimidated by the idea, as if working with their thoughts and emotions somehow invalidates the very real physical pain they experience. Others associate these methods with stigma, thinking, *It's not all in my head*, or assume that techniques like mindfulness or visualization won't make a meaningful difference.

These concerns are valid, especially for those who have spent years searching for answers. But psychological tools aren't about denying pain or suggesting it's imagined. They are about teaching the brain new ways to respond to pain signals—physically rewiring pain pathways in a way that reduces suffering. Far from being "woo-woo," these techniques are backed by decades of neuroscience showing how they calm the nervous system, reduce inflammation, and help the body regulate pain more effectively.

If the idea of trying these tools feels overwhelming or unfamiliar, start small. Think of them as experiments—ways to gently test what might help you feel a little better, one step at a time. Later in this book, we'll explore practical ways to integrate these techniques into daily life, from breathwork to cognitive reframing.

For now, just remember healing isn't about working harder. It's about working *smarter*—using the brain's natural ability to change as a foundation for resilience and recovery.

SIDEBAR

Take Action: Moving Beyond Judgement

Take two minutes to observe your pain without judgment. Sit quietly and note its qualities (e.g., sharp, dull, constant, or intermittent).

Remind yourself: *This is a moment of discomfort, but I don't have to fight it.*

REWIRING THE BRAIN: THE SCIENCE BEHIND PSYCHOLOGICAL RESILIENCE

For most of his life, Andre had relied on his body. He was a competitive soccer player, training six days a week, pushing through injuries, and living by the motto "no pain, no gain." In his early twenties, he was on the verge of playing professionally, with scouts watching his every game. But a lower back injury—what seemed like just another strain at first—refused to heal.

At first, Andre did what he had always done: he trained through it. Pain was just part of the sport, something to grit his teeth through. His coaches had drilled into him that stopping meant weakness. He went through rounds of physical therapy, cortisone injections, and painkillers, trying to get back on the field. But instead of healing, the pain became a constant presence. When it became clear that his body wouldn't let him play at the level he once had, Andre had to walk away from the sport that had defined him.

The years that followed were filled with frustration. Without soccer, his body—once his greatest asset—felt like his enemy. The pain was unpredictable; some days it was manageable, other days it flared out of nowhere, leaving him exhausted and defeated. He tried every available treatment: more physical therapy, medications, even surgery. Each approach promised relief, but the pain always returned.

His endurance mindset didn't translate to recovery. For years, he had been conditioned to believe that pushing through was the answer. But chronic pain wasn't like a tough game—it didn't reward resilience in the way he had always understood it. No amount of gritting his teeth made it better.

His psychologist explained something Andre had never considered: his brain had built deep pathways linking pain with fear, frustration, and helplessness. The pain itself was real—but the way his brain processed it had been reshaped over years of endurance thinking. His brain was reinforcing pain patterns, keeping his nervous system in a constant state of high alert.

Skeptical but curious, he began to try mindfulness exercises. The next time his pain flared, instead of immediately tightening against it, he paused. He took a slow breath and told himself: this is discomfort, but I don't have to fight it.

It felt unnatural at first—like trying to unlearn years of instinct. But something shifted. The pain didn't magically disappear, but he didn't spiral the way he usually did. That tiny bit of space—between the pain and his emotional reaction—was new.

Over time, he started calling his pain background noise instead of a constant battle. The difference was subtle but profound—he wasn't bracing against every sensation. He wasn't pushing through or ignoring it, but he also wasn't letting it consume him.

He began integrating other techniques: breathing exercises, brief meditations, catching negative thought loops before they spiraled. For the first time in years, he saw that pain wasn't just something to endure—it was something his brain could retrain itself to manage.

Like Andre, you have the ability to reshape how your brain processes pain. It starts with small steps. Let's explore the science behind some of the most powerful techniques.

RECLAIMING CONTROL: YOUR PATH FORWARD

At this point, you may be wondering: What does all of this mean for me? Understanding the psychological systems that sustain chronic pain is one thing but applying that knowledge to your own experience is another. If you've lived with pain for months or years, it's understandable to feel skeptical—perhaps even exhausted—by the idea of trying yet another approach. But what if this isn't about trying harder? What if it's about trying differently?

Andre's story is not unique. As doctors specializing in pain and resilience, we've worked with hundreds of patients who, like Andre, had exhausted every physical intervention and were left with the sinking feeling that nothing would ever change. But the truth is, while chronic pain does reshape the brain, the brain is not fixed. Neuroplasticity, the very process that amplifies pain over time, can also be harnessed to rewire those patterns in a healthier direction.

Your journey forward does not require ignoring your pain or pretending it doesn't exist. Instead, it asks you to approach it differently—to train your nervous system to respond in ways that reduce suffering rather than reinforcing it.

Let's explore a few foundational strategies.

Mindfulness: Training Your Brain to Focus on the Present

Andre had spent years pushing through pain, keeping his focus on the next game, the next goal, the next stretch of endurance. But when his pain became chronic, that approach stopped working. His thoughts spiraled—anticipating pain, bracing against it, fearing its return. His pain wasn't just physical; it had become mental, shaping his every decision and reaction.

Mindfulness changed that. Unlike the strategies he had relied on before, mindfulness didn't ask him to push harder or fight through. Instead, it asked him to do something that felt almost impossible: to stop, observe, and allow.

Mindfulness is the practice of paying attention to the present moment with curiosity and without judgment. In the context of chronic pain, this means observing pain without immediately reacting to it with fear or frustration. When you notice pain and allow yourself to acknowledge it without bracing against it, you activate different brain pathways—ones that can help regulate pain instead of amplifying it.

Neuroscience research has shown that mindfulness doesn't just reduce the emotional toll of pain—it physically changes the brain. Studies using fMRI scans reveal that long-term mindfulness practice strengthens the prefrontal cortex, the part of the brain responsible for emotional regulation. At the same time, mindfulness decreases activity in the amygdala, calming the body's stress response. It also quiets the default mode network, the system responsible for repetitive, distressing thoughts about pain.

This shift is profound. Over time, mindfulness can reduce pain's intensity, not by eliminating it, but by changing how the brain interprets it.

Try It: A Mindfulness Exercise for Pain Management

1. Find a quiet place. Sit or lie down comfortably. Close your eyes if that feels comfortable.
2. Notice your breathing. Without changing anything, observe the natural rhythm of your inhale and exhale.
3. Scan your body. Bring awareness to different areas of your body. Notice where tension or discomfort exists.
4. Acknowledge pain without judgment. If you feel pain, observe it without immediately reacting. Instead of thinking "This is awful," try saying, "This is a sensation. I am noticing it, but I do not have to fight it."
5. Gently return to your breath. If your mind wanders, guide it back to your breath.

Reflection Questions

- How do you typically respond to pain—by bracing, ignoring, or reacting emotionally?

- What did you notice when you observed your pain without judgment?

- Could practicing mindfulness during pain episodes change how you experience them?

Cognitive Reframing: Shifting Negative Thought Patterns

When Andre first learned about cognitive reframing, he dismissed it. "Changing my thoughts won't change my pain," he thought. But his psychologist explained something that stuck with him: your thoughts are messages to your brain. If they reinforce fear and helplessness, your brain amplifies the pain response. If they signal resilience and control, your brain learns a new way to respond.

Cognitive reframing is the process of identifying unhelpful thoughts and replacing them with more constructive alternatives. It's not about denying pain—it's about shifting your relationship with it.

Imagine you wake up with a flare-up. Your immediate thought might be: "This pain will never end." Now, imagine shifting that thought slightly:

"This is a tough moment, but I have tools to get through it."

Research shows that reframing reduces activity in the amygdala while strengthening the prefrontal cortex, improving emotional regulation. Studies have also linked cognitive reframing to lower cortisol levels, meaning less stress and inflammation—both of which can worsen pain.

Try It: Reframing Your Pain Narrative

1. Write down one negative thought you frequently have about pain. (Example: "This pain is ruining my life.")
2. Ask yourself: Is this an absolute truth, or is it a reaction? (Example: "Is pain ruining my entire life, or is it making some things harder?")
3. Reframe it into a more constructive statement. (Example: "This pain is hard, but I am learning how to manage it.")

Reflection Questions

- What are some common negative thoughts you have about pain?
- How do those thoughts influence your emotions and body?
- What is one thought you could start reframing today?

Visualization: Changing How Your Brain Interprets Pain

The brain doesn't just passively receive pain signals—it interprets them. This is why some people experience severe pain from a minor injury, while others can undergo surgery with minimal discomfort. How the brain processes pain is just as important as the pain itself.

One powerful way to influence this process is visualization. This practice uses mental imagery to alter how the brain perceives pain, engaging the sensory cortex in a way that reduces its intensity.

Scientific studies on guided imagery show that visualization exercises can reduce activity in pain-processing areas of the brain. Athletes use visualization to speed up injury recovery, and cancer patients use it to manage chemotherapy side effects. The same principles apply to chronic pain.

Try It: Visualization for Pain Relief

1. Close your eyes and take a deep breath. Picture your pain as a shape, color, or object in your body. Maybe it's a tight knot, a burning flame, or a heavy stone.
2. Now, imagine transforming it.
    - If your pain is a jagged rock, smooth it out.
    - If it's a burning flame, picture it cooling down.
    - If it's a heavy weight, imagine it getting lighter.

3. Breathe into the change. As you inhale, see the painful sensation shrinking. As you exhale, release tension.

Reflection Questions

- What did your pain look like in your mind? Did it shift during the exercise?
- How did your body feel afterward?
- Could you practice this when pain flares to change its intensity?

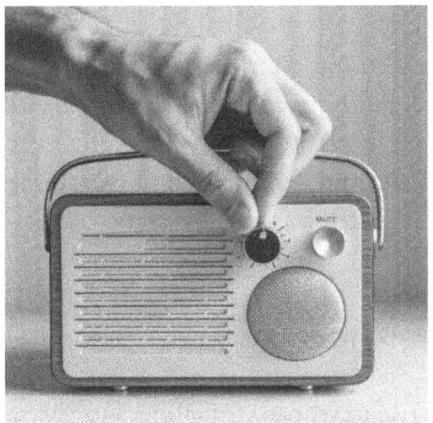

Picture your pain as a glowing dial. Imagine yourself reaching out and turning the dial down, noticing how your body start to relax with each turn. How does this feel?

Emotional Regulation: Building Resilience Through Self-Compassion and Gratitude

Emotional regulation is the ability to manage stress, frustration, and distress in a way that doesn't amplify pain. Many people with chronic pain experience heightened emotional responses—understandably so. But research shows that unchecked emotions can actually reinforce pain pathways, strengthening the pain response over time.

Two powerful techniques for emotional regulation are self-compassion and gratitude.

Self-Compassion: Talking to Yourself Like a Friend

Many people with chronic pain blame themselves for their suffering. They feel frustrated, guilty, or ashamed for not "handling it better." But self-criticism only increases stress, making pain worse. Self-compassion, on the other hand, activates oxytocin and dopamine—neurochemicals that reduce pain and increase a sense of safety.

Try It: Practicing Self-Compassion

1. Think of a friend who is struggling. How would you comfort them?
2. Now, turn that kindness toward yourself. Instead of thinking "I should be stronger," try "I'm doing my best, and that's enough."

Gratitude: A Simple Practice with Big Results

Gratitude isn't about ignoring pain—it's about training the brain to notice what else exists alongside it. Studies show that gratitude increases activity in the prefrontal cortex, helping shift focus away from distress.

Try It: A 3-Minute Gratitude Exercise

1. Write down three things you're grateful for today, no matter how small.
2. Reflect on how those things bring comfort, joy, or relief.
3. Notice if your mood shifts, even slightly.

Reflection Questions

- How does your inner dialogue affect your pain?
- What is one way you can practice self-compassion today?
- How might focusing on small positives help rewire your brain's pain response?

Many people who live with chronic pain feel overwhelmed by the idea of change. But rewiring the brain is not about making one massive transformation—it's about making small, sustainable shifts over time. As doctors who have guided patients through this process, we have seen firsthand that even simple daily practices can create profound changes.

As you finish this chapter, consider one small step you could take today to start reshaping your relationship with pain. Maybe it's practicing deep breathing for two minutes. Maybe it's pausing to notice your first emotional reaction to pain. Maybe it's reframing just one thought. Whatever it is, remember: Small steps, repeated over time, can create lasting change.

LOOKING AHEAD: PAIN, MEDICATIONS, AND THE BRAIN'S NATURAL HEALING SYSTEMS

We've established that your brain is not fixed—it's constantly changing and adapting based on your experiences. This ability, known as neuroplasticity, is what makes it possible to rewire your brain and reshape how it processes pain. Psychological resilience is the key to unlocking this potential, using tools like mindfulness, cognitive reframing, visualization, and emotional regulation to reduce pain's grip and restore balance to your body and mind.

But psychological tools are not the only factor in pain management, nor are they a replacement for medical treatment. Many people living with chronic pain turn to medications—particularly opioids—in an attempt to regain control over their discomfort. For acute injuries, opioids can be a necessary and effective tool, but in chronic pain, they often change how the brain processes pain over time, sometimes making it more difficult for the body to regulate pain naturally.

This is where the next phase of pain management comes in: understanding how medications affect the brain's pain systems and how we can work with the brain's own mu-opioid system to enhance natural pain relief mechanisms. In the next chapter, we'll explore:

- Why opioids often fail to provide lasting relief in chronic pain and how they can contribute to increased pain sensitivity over time.
- The brain's natural pain relief system (the mu-opioid system) and how resilience-based strategies can reactivate it.
- Pain reprocessing therapy, an emerging approach designed to help the brain reinterpret pain signals as non-threatening.
- The placebo and nocebo effects, and how our beliefs about pain can shape our experience of it—for better or worse.
- How breaking the pain-stress loop allows the nervous system to return to a calmer, more balanced state.

The brain has remarkable built-in tools for managing pain, but chronic pain can block or weaken those mechanisms. By understanding how both medications and psychological approaches impact the nervous system, we can develop a more comprehensive, sustainable strategy for becoming resilient.

CHAPTER 7
THE PAIN-STRESS FEEDBACK LOOP

Andre had made progress. The tools he learned in therapy—mindfulness, cognitive reframing, and visualization—had started to shift the way he experienced pain. He no longer felt as controlled by it as he once had. But some days, the pain still got the better of him. It wasn't just the physical discomfort; it was the exhaustion, the unpredictability, the way it stole his focus and drained his energy.

Then there were the setbacks. A bad flare-up could unravel weeks of progress, leaving him questioning whether anything he was doing was actually working. And when that happened, his stress skyrocketed. His body tensed. His breathing shortened. His mind spiraled back into old patterns of frustration: *What if this never gets better? What if I'm just fooling myself?*

After a particularly rough stretch, he brought his concerns to his doctor. "I don't get it," Andre admitted. "I do everything right. I manage my triggers, I take care of my body. But I still have these flare-ups, and when they hit, they take over everything. It's like my pain has a mind of its own."

His doctor nodded. "You've been working on your physical recovery and learning how to reframe your pain. That's great. But let me ask you

—what's happening in your mind *before* these flare-ups? Not just when they start, but in the hours or even days leading up to them?"

Andre frowned. "I don't know. I guess I get stressed. Sometimes I'm already on edge before the pain starts."

"That's what I suspected," the doctor said. "Pain doesn't just come from one place. The biopsychosocial model tells us that pain has three major components—biological, psychological, and social. Right now, you're managing the biological side with physical therapy and exercise. You're learning to navigate the social side by staying engaged instead of withdrawing. But psychologically? That's still your weak link."

Andre absorbed the words. Despite everything he had learned about mindfulness, brain chemistry, and how the default mode network fuels negative thought loops, he still instinctively blamed his worst pain days on his body—on something he had done wrong or something that wasn't healing properly. But what if his mind was playing an even bigger role than he realized?

It wasn't that the pain was imaginary—far from it. The brain doesn't just interpret pain; it can amplify it by triggering real, physiological responses. When Andre became stressed or fearful, his brain sent signals to release cortisol and activate the fight-or-flight system. That, in turn, tensed his muscles, disrupted his breathing, and made his nervous system more sensitive to pain. His psychological stress was creating a biological storm.

His doctor continued. "For some people, the biggest driver of pain is structural—damaged tissue, inflammation, or nerve dysfunction. For others, it's loneliness or lack of support. But in your case? Your pain-stress feedback loop is being driven by psychological factors more than anything. When you feel stressed or fearful about pain, your nervous system reacts by making it worse. And once you're in that cycle, it's hard to break out."

It made sense. The more he feared the next flare-up, the more likely it seemed to happen. The more exhausted he became, the harder it was to cope. The more he worried about how much pain he'd be in tomorrow, the worse he felt today.

Andre took a deep breath. "So, what do I do?"

His doctor smiled. "You've already started. The fact that you recognize this pattern is huge. Now, the next step is learning how to *interrupt* it before it spirals. You need strategies to regulate your nervous system—to catch stress before it fuels your pain."

Andre thought back to his training days as an athlete. He had always relied on his physical endurance to push through pain. Now, he needed to build his psychological endurance—not by gritting his teeth and ignoring stress, but by actively working to break the cycle before it started.

This was the next phase of his recovery: learning how to calm his nervous system, shift his mindset, and stop stress from amplifying his pain.

THE EMOTIONAL TOLL OF THE PAIN-STRESS LOOP

Pain is not just a signal; it's a threat detector. When you feel pain, your amygdala, the brain's alarm system, reacts as though you're in danger. It floods your system with stress hormones like cortisol and adrenaline, priming your body to fight, flee, or freeze. This response is critical in moments of actual danger—if you break a bone, your body wants you to stop moving and protect the injury.

But in chronic pain, this alarm system doesn't shut off. The brain stays on high alert, even when there's no immediate danger. The result? Persistent muscle tension, restricted blood flow, and heightened inflammation—all of which make pain feel even worse.

As we've talked about in earlier chapters, it's easy to get caught in a feedback loop, pain causing stress and stress worsening pain. For Andre, this meant that on days when he worried about pain, his body braced for it before it even arrived. His breathing became shallow, his muscles tensed, his mind fixated on every twinge. The more stress he felt, the more his body responded with pain.

Stress isn't just emotional; it has physiological consequences that reinforce pain. When stress levels are high, the brain's default mode network (DMN) becomes more active. This is the same network responsible for self-reflection, and when pain is involved, it can become a loop of negative thoughts:

"This pain will never end."

"I can't handle this."

"I'm broken."

Research has shown that chronic pain keeps the DMN stuck in these loops, amplifying distress. One study published in *Nature Neuroscience* found that people with chronic pain showed increased DMN activity compared to those without pain, meaning their brains were reinforcing pain-related thought patterns without conscious effort.

At the same time, prolonged stress disrupts the body's hormonal and immune systems. Elevated cortisol levels make it harder for the body to regulate inflammation, while chronic stress weakens immune function, slowing recovery and making pain flare-ups more frequent. The longer this cycle continues, the harder it is to break.

Andre had always thought of himself as mentally tough. Soccer had trained him to endure discomfort, to push through fatigue, to perform under pressure. But chronic pain was different. It wasn't something he could outwork or push past. Over time, his confidence eroded. His pain wasn't just physical anymore—it carried frustration, grief, and fear.

This is the emotional toll of chronic pain. The constant stress makes anxiety spike, leading to hypervigilance about every sensation. Depression sets in when pain limits daily life, making it feel like the future is shrinking. These emotions don't just accompany pain—they shape how the brain processes it, strengthening pain pathways in a way that makes even mild discomfort feel unbearable.

Andre began to see that his body wasn't just reacting to pain—it was reacting to the stress and fear surrounding it. If he could interrupt that stress response, he might be able to interrupt the pain itself. But how?

This is why Breaking the pain-stress loop requires addressing both the mind and body. But trust us when we say that the pain-stress cycle *can be interrupted*. We've done just that with countless patients by addressing their chronic pain at the whole-body level through attention on all three areas of the biopsychosocial model. After beginning to get your bodily systems rebalanced as we talked about in Part One, by then calming the nervous system and shifting your brain's focus, you can reduce stress and lessen its impact on pain.

Mindfulness and visualization help deactivate the amygdala, reducing its alarm signals and helping you gain more control over your pain responses.

Relaxation techniques like progressive muscle relaxation or deep breathing counteract muscle tension and restore blood flow, reducing physical discomfort.

Cognitive reframing disrupts the DMN's negative thought cycles, replacing fear-based patterns with more constructive ones.

For Andre, like most of our patients, the shift happened gradually. He started by noticing when he was holding his breath or tensing his muscles before the pain even hit. Instead of clenching through it, he practiced deep breathing. He experimented with visualization, imagining his pain shrinking like a dimming light. He worked on catching negative thoughts before they spiraled.

By working consistently with the below tools, he made steady, empowering progress, beginning to get both the physical and psychological manifestations of his chronic pain under his control and developing resiliency to prevent the pain from ever taking hold over his as aggressively as it had before again.

Before looking at these tools in-depth, let's back up a moment.

Andre wanted to believe that if he could calm his nervous system, his pain would start to ease. But a part of him was skeptical. If chronic pain was so deeply wired into his brain, could simple techniques like breathing or reframing his thoughts really make a difference?

He wasn't alone in this doubt. Many chronic pain patients, searching for real relief, turn to medications—especially opioids—as their primary solution. After all, opioids are prescribed as some of the strongest painkillers available. For a time, Andre had gone down that road, too. His doctors in the past when he was playing soccer had told him that pain was something to be "managed," and medication seemed like the only tool he had left.

But over time, he found himself needing more—more pills, more doses, more hope that the next refill would finally bring him relief. Instead, his body only felt more tangled in the pain. What he didn't realize then was that opioids weren't just failing to fix his pain—they were making it worse.

SAHAR SWIDAN & MATTHEW BENNETT

WHY OPIOIDS OFTEN FAIL FOR CHRONIC PAIN

For years, doctors were taught that opioids were the most effective treatment for pain. In cases of acute pain—such as post-surgical recovery or injury—these medications can provide critical relief. But when it comes to chronic pain, opioids often fail to deliver long-term results.

Andre learned this firsthand. When his back pain persisted after he left soccer, his doctor prescribed an opioid to help him manage it. At first, it worked—his pain dulled, and for a while, he felt like he had some control over it. But over time, the relief faded. The pain returned sooner between doses, forcing him to take more just to keep functioning. His doctor increased the dosage. When that wasn't enough, he switched to a stronger prescription.

It wasn't until years later, sitting in that pain psychologist's office, that Andre fully understood what had happened. His brain had adapted to the medication, requiring higher and higher doses to achieve the same effect—a process called tolerance. And as he continued taking opioids, his body's natural pain regulation system had weakened.

What Andre didn't know then was that long-term opioid use suppresses the brain's mu-opioid system, which is responsible for producing endorphins—our body's built-in painkillers. Over time, opioids don't just change how the brain processes pain; they can actually make pain worse. Research shows that prolonged opioid use activates immune-like cells in the brain called glial cells, which release inflammatory signals. This means that rather than reducing pain, long-term opioid use can increase inflammation in the nervous system, making the pain feel sharper and more persistent.

So why did his doctors prescribe opioids in the first place?

For decades, medical providers have been trained to treat pain primarily as a biological issue—a matter of tissue damage, nerves, and inflammation. The assumption was that if someone was in pain, it must mean there was an injury or dysfunction that needed to be "fixed." Pharmaceutical companies reinforced this belief, aggressively marketing opioids as a safe and effective solution. Many doctors genuinely wanted to help their patients, and with few alternative treatments being taught in medical school, opioids became the go-to option for chronic pain.

But as research on chronic pain evolved, it became clear that opioids were not only ineffective for long-term pain management but also potentially harmful. Studies showed that they did little to address the underlying mechanisms of chronic pain and often left patients worse off—physically dependent on medication while still experiencing significant discomfort.

UNLOCKING THE BRAIN'S NATURAL PAIN-RELIEF SYSTEM

The thing that Andre, like most of our patients, never realized is that while he had Andre spent years relying on medication to manage his pain, his brain already had its own built-in pain relief system—the mu-opioid system. This system releases endorphins, the body's natural painkillers, which help regulate discomfort and create a sense of well-being.

But after prolonged opioid use and years of chronic pain, Andre's brain had stopped using this system effectively. His body had learned to expect relief from medication rather than activating its own internal pain-relief mechanisms. The good news? Just as the brain can become dependent on external opioids, it can also be trained to reactivate its natural pain-relief pathways.

One of the simplest ways to do this is through mindfulness. Studies show that mindfulness meditation increases the brain's production of endorphins, engaging the mu-opioid system and reducing pain perception. When Andre began practicing mindfulness, he noticed that his pain didn't disappear—but it felt less overwhelming. His body became less reactive to discomfort, and he could engage in daily activities with less fear.

Gratitude practices also helped. At first, Andre dismissed the idea of keeping a gratitude journal—it felt too simple to have any real impact. But neuroscience research suggests otherwise. Reflecting on what we're grateful for activates the brain's reward pathways, which are closely linked to the mu-opioid system. This shift in focus—from pain to appreciation—helped Andre's brain move away from its constant cycle of distress.

Similarly, cognitive reframing allowed Andre to take control of his pain narrative. When he replaced fear-based thoughts like *I can't handle this* with *I'm learning to manage this,* his brain responded differently. Instead of triggering a stress response, these new thoughts signaled safety, reducing pain's intensity.

Andre wasn't just managing pain anymore—he was rewiring his brain's response to it.

REWIRING THE BRAIN WITH PAIN REPROCESSING THERAPY

As Andre continued exploring new approaches to pain management, we introduced him to a method called pain reprocessing therapy (PRT). Grounded in the principles of neuroplasticity, PRT is designed to retrain the brain to interpret pain signals differently.

In chronic pain, the brain often misinterprets signals from the body as dangerous, even when no real harm is present. This constant state of alarm keeps pain pathways active, reinforcing discomfort. PRT works by helping patients recognize that many of their pain signals are not a sign of actual damage but rather a learned response from the brain.

A groundbreaking study published in *JAMA Psychiatry* found that 66% of participants who underwent PRT reported being nearly or completely pain-free after just four weeks. Brain imaging confirmed reduced activity in pain-processing regions of the brain, supporting the idea that PRT doesn't just mask pain—it rewires how the brain interprets it.

For Andre, this approach changed everything. Working alongside his pain psychologist, we had him identify moments when he was unconsciously bracing against pain—tensing his body, holding his breath, catastrophizing about future discomfort. Instead of reacting with fear, he practiced responding with curiosity: *Is this pain actually dangerous? Is my body really in harm's way?*

Slowly, his brain began to process pain differently. His flare-ups became less intense. His stress response weakened. He still had pain, but it no longer dictated his every move.

PRT aligned with everything he had been learning—about mindfulness, cognitive reframing, and visualization. These weren't just psychological techniques; they were tools for physically reshaping his brain's pain pathways.

That shift in perspective changed everything. Over time, Andre worked on shifting his thoughts, learning how cognitive reframing could help calm his body's alarm system. Each step wasn't just about reducing pain; it was about building resilience.

Here's how you can begin doing the same.

BREAKING THE LOOP: TOOLS FOR CALMING THE NERVOUS SYSTEM

1. Progressive Muscle Relaxation (PMR): Releasing Tension from Head to Toe

Muscle tension often builds up unnoticed in response to pain and stress, keeping the body in a defensive state. Progressive muscle relaxation (PMR) is a technique that helps release stored tension, signaling to the nervous system that it's safe to relax.

How to practice:

- Find a quiet, comfortable space where you won't be disturbed. Lie down or sit in a supported position.
- Take a slow, deep breath in. As you exhale, notice any tension in your body.
- Begin at your feet: Tense the muscles in your toes and feet for five seconds, squeezing gently but firmly. Then, release the tension completely and feel the difference.
- Move up to your calves: Tense for five seconds, then release.
- Continue this process with your thighs, stomach, chest, shoulders, arms, hands, jaw, and forehead, spending a few moments relaxing each area after tensing.

- Once you've scanned your whole body, take three deep breaths and notice how your muscles feel.

Journaling reflection:

- After completing this exercise, how does your body feel compared to before?
- Did you notice any areas of chronic tension? How might pain be influencing those areas?
- Could you use this practice at night to improve sleep or during stressful moments to release tension?

2. Deep Breathing for Stress Relief: Resetting the Nervous System

When you experience stress or pain, your breathing naturally becomes shallow and rapid. This signals danger to the nervous system, reinforcing the pain-stress loop. Practicing slow, controlled breathing can shift your body from a stress response to a state of relaxation.

How to practice:

- Sit comfortably, placing one hand on your belly and the other on your chest.
- Inhale deeply through your nose for four counts, feeling your belly rise (not just your chest).
- Hold your breath for four counts, allowing the air to settle.
- Exhale slowly through your mouth for six counts, letting go of tension as you breathe out.
- Repeat this cycle for one to three minutes, focusing on making your exhale slightly longer than your inhale.

Try this variation: Box breathing

If your mind feels especially restless, try box breathing, a technique used by athletes and military personnel to stay calm under pressure.

- Inhale for four counts
- Hold for four counts
- Exhale for four counts
- Hold for four counts
- Repeat for five to ten cycles

Journaling reflection:

- How does your body feel after practicing this breathwork?
- Did any particular thoughts or emotions arise?
- Could you incorporate this into your daily routine (e.g., upon waking, before bed, or when pain flares)?

3. Breaking Negative Thought Loops: Reframing Pain Narratives

The way we think about pain impacts how we experience it. Negative thought patterns, like "I'll never get better" or "I can't handle this pain," can reinforce distress and strengthen pain pathways in the brain. Cognitive reframing helps shift these thoughts, weakening their grip and opening space for more helpful beliefs.

How to practice:

- Identify a recurring negative thought you have about pain. Write it down.
- Ask yourself: Is this thought an absolute truth, or is it an emotional reaction?
- Rewrite the thought in a more balanced way. Here are some examples:
    - Instead of: "This pain is ruining my life."

- Try: "This pain is challenging, but I'm learning new ways to manage it."
  - Instead of: "I'm broken."
    - Try: "My body is struggling, but it is also adapting and healing."
  - Instead of: "Nothing ever works for me."
    - Try: "I am still exploring what works. Some strategies take time to show results."

Journaling reflection:

- What negative thoughts come up most often when your pain flares?
- How do these thoughts influence your emotions and body?
- What is one belief about your pain that you could reframe?

4. Visualization Exercise: Changing Your Pain Perception

Your brain processes pain partly through mental imagery. Studies show that visualization can alter how the brain interprets pain, making it feel less intense. This exercise helps retrain your sensory cortex to downregulate pain perception.

How to practice:

- Close your eyes and take a few deep breaths. Imagine your pain as a shape in your body—perhaps a heavy stone in your lower back or a tight knot in your neck.
- Now, picture that shape softening, shrinking, or changing color. If it's jagged, smooth it out. If it's fiery red, let it cool to a soft blue.
- Visualize warmth and healing energy surrounding the painful area, gently easing tension and discomfort.
- After a few minutes, take a deep breath and open your eyes.

Journaling reflection:

- What did your pain look like in your mind? Did it shift during the exercise?
- How did your body feel after the visualization?
- Could you practice this when pain flares to help regulate its intensity?

RESILIENCE AND THE BRAIN: BUILDING NEW PATHWAYS

Building psychological resilience around pain, as we've seen, isn't about instant fixes or sweeping changes; it's about creating new pathways in the brain, one small step at a time. Through the process of neuroplasticity, each mindful breath, reframed thought, or moment of gratitude helps rewire your brain, making it less reactive to pain and more capable of balance and recovery. These changes don't happen overnight, but with consistent effort, they create long-term progress that ripples throughout your entire body.

In the name of reducing a problem into smaller parts in order to better meet it head on, let's look at several small things you can carry forward to practice steadily building your resilience.

THE POWER OF MICRO-WINS

Resilience often starts with "micro-wins"—small, manageable actions that shift the brain in a healthier direction. Think of it like planting seeds. Each moment you focus on the present instead of pain or reframe a negative thought into a more empowering one, you're nurturing pathways in your brain that promote calm and control. Over time, these small victories add up, creating profound and lasting changes in how your brain processes pain.

For example, practicing mindfulness for just two minutes a day might feel insignificant at first, but research shows that even brief mindfulness practices can reduce activity in the amygdala and strengthen the prefrontal cortex. Similarly, expressing gratitude once a day can help quiet the default mode network (DMN), reducing rumination and fostering emotional balance. These practices are like daily deposits in a resilience bank account—the more you invest, the stronger your foundation becomes.

SIDEBAR

Take Action: The Power of Resilience Deposits

What's one small action—a micro-win—you can take today to begin rewiring your brain for resilience? How might this ripple into other areas of your life over time?

THE RIPPLE EFFECT OF RESILIENCE

Changes in the brain don't exist in isolation; they have cascading effects throughout your body. When you calm your brain's alarm system, you also calm your nervous system, shifting from a state of "fight or flight" to "rest and repair." This supports the endocrine system by lowering stress hormones like cortisol, which in turn helps regulate inflammation and promotes healing.

At the same time, resilience-building practices improve immune system function, allowing your body to focus on recovery instead of constantly managing stress. This ripple effect shows why psychological resilience isn't just a mental exercise—it's a holistic process that transforms how you feel, think, and function.

The path to resilience is not linear. Some days will feel easier than others, and that's okay. What matters most is consistency. Each small effort—whether it's taking a moment to breathe deeply during a stressful situation or writing down one thing you're grateful for—contributes to long-term healing.

Over time, these practices change the brain's default state. Instead of being stuck in fear, stress, or pain, your brain begins to anchor itself in calm, focus, and hope. This doesn't mean the pain disappears completely, but it does mean you'll have the tools and the strength to respond to it in a way that's less consuming and more empowering. The very same neuroplasticity that once reinforced pain can now be used to help you reclaim your life. By calming your mind, reframing your thoughts, and engaging in simple, consistent practices, you have the power to reshape your brain's response to pain and build a foundation for healing.

We hope this chapter has not only shown you the science behind these tools but also helped ease any hesitation you may have felt about using them. These aren't "soft" approaches—they're powerful, evidence-based methods rooted in the way your brain and body work. If you've ever felt unsure about trying mindfulness, visualization, or reframing, we encourage you to take that first small step. The journey begins with one breath, one thought, one choice.

As you move forward, imagine what it might feel like to experience a little less fear, a little more clarity, and a greater sense of control. Imagine being able to respond to pain with calm instead of panic, to focus on what matters most, and to reconnect with the parts of yourself that chronic pain may have taken away.

Psychological resilience is only one part of the story. To thrive beyond pain, we also need connection—support from others who understand us, relationships that lift us up, and a sense of belonging. In the next chapter, we'll explore the social dimension of resilience: how chronic pain affects relationships and how rebuilding connection can create a powerful buffer against stress and pain. Together, these tools form the foundation for a life of greater balance, meaning, and joy.

Resilience doesn't stop with the brain. It extends to the relationships you nurture, the purpose you find, and the way you engage with the world around you. In the next chapter, we'll explore how social connections can play a pivotal role in building resilience, buffering stress, and helping you thrive beyond pain.

In the next part of the book, we'll look closer at how pain affects the third circle of the biopsychosocial model: our lives as social creatures.

CHAPTER-END ACTIVITY

Practical Strategies for Psychological Resilience

Building resilience doesn't require perfection or massive changes all at once. Instead, it's about small, consistent practices that fit into your daily life. These practices can be tailored to your needs and preferences, creating a toolkit that evolves with you. In this section, we'll preview some practical strategies that will be explored in more detail later in the book.

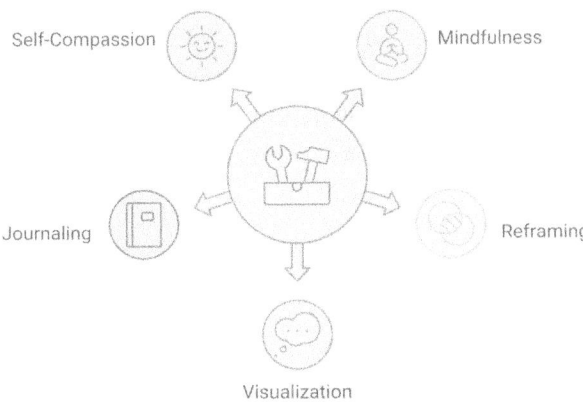

Resilience Toolkit

Mindfulness as a Foundation

Mindfulness is one of the most effective tools for calming the nervous system and rewiring the brain. Simply focusing on your breath for two minutes a day can start to reduce activity in the amygdala and shift your body into a "rest and repair" mode. Over time, these moments of calm help build resilience to stress and pain.

Cognitive Reframing for Mental Strength

Negative thoughts like *I can't handle this pain,* or *Nothing will ever change* can reinforce pain pathways in the brain. Cognitive reframing helps you challenge these thoughts and replace them with more balanced ones, such as *This is tough, but I'm learning how to manage it* or *I've gotten through hard moments before, and I can do it again.* This practice strengthens the prefrontal cortex, improving emotional regulation and creating a more hopeful mindset.

Visualization to Shift Perception

Visualization techniques, like imagining your pain as a glowing dial and mentally turning it down, can help reduce the intensity of pain signals in the brain. These exercises work by retraining the sensory cortex to interpret pain in a less threatening way, creating a sense of control over your experience.

Journaling for Emotional Balance

Writing down your thoughts and emotions can be a powerful way to process frustration, sadness, or anger associated with chronic pain. Journaling also helps you identify patterns in your thinking and behavior, making it easier to recognize and reframe negative loops. A simple gratitude journal—where you list three things you're grateful for each day—can quiet the default mode network and build a foundation of positivity.

Self-Compassion as a Daily Practice

Chronic pain can make you feel isolated or frustrated with yourself. Self-compassion involves treating yourself with the same kindness you'd offer to a friend in need. This practice reduces emotional distress, quiets the DMN, and fosters a sense of resilience. For example, when pain flares, try saying to yourself, *This is hard, but I'm doing my best.*

Start Small and Stay Consistent

You don't need to do all of these practices at once. In fact, trying to take on too much can feel overwhelming. Start with one or two strategies that resonate with you and commit to practicing them consistently. If your energy is low, even small actions—like 30 seconds of mindful breathing or writing down just one thing you're grateful for—can create meaningful change over time.

Which of these strategies feels most approachable for you to try? How might it fit into your daily routine?

To make these strategies a reality, use our weekly resilience tracker in the following activity.

CHAPTER-END ACTIVITY

Your Weekly Resilience Tracker

This tracker is designed to help you build resilience one step at a time. Each day, choose 1–3 activities that feel manageable. There's no need to do everything—focus on small wins and celebrate your consistency.

Day	Mindfulness	Reframing Negative Thoughts	Visualization	Journaling	Self-Compassion Practice
Monday	2 minutes focusing on your breath	Reframe one thought about pain	Visualize turning down pain dial	Write 3 things you're grateful for	Say, *I'm doing my best today*
Tuesday	5 minutes noticing your surroundings	Replace *I can't handle this* with *I'm learning to manage*	Imagine pain fading into the distance	Write about a moment that made you smile	Treat yourself to something comforting
Wednesday	3 minutes of body scanning	Identify one helpful belief to repeat	Picture yourself relaxed and at ease	Reflect on one thing you're proud of	Say, *This is hard, but I'm trying my best*
Thursday	2 minutes of mindful walking	Reframe a frustration as a growth opportunity	Imagine your body healing itself	Write about a challenge you overcame	Place your hand on your heart and breathe deeply
Friday	5 minutes observing your breath	Write one empowering thought	Visualize calm waves washing over you	List 3 things you accomplished this week	Say, *I am worthy of care and kindness*
Saturday	Practice mindful eating during one meal	Replace *Nothing will ever change* with *Small steps lead to progress*	Imagine pain shrinking in size	Free-write for 5 minutes about your feelings	Spend 5 minutes doing something just for you
Sunday	Reflect on the week with gratitude	Repeat one positive thought that resonated with you	Picture a future moment of joy	Write about how you felt after practicing resilience this week	Rest without guilt—acknowledge your efforts

How to Use the Tracker:

Daily Check-In: At the end of each day, reflect on which activities you completed and how they made you feel.

Celebrate Consistency: The goal isn't perfection. Even one small action a day is a step toward building resilience.

Adjust as Needed: This tracker is a guide, not a rulebook. Feel free to modify it to fit your needs and energy levels.

CHAPTER 8
HOW TRAUMA AMPLIFIES CHRONIC PAIN

Andre never thought much about trauma. He had a solid upbringing—his family wasn't perfect, but whose was? He grew up playing high-level soccer, which had taught him discipline, teamwork, and how to push through pain. He had always assumed that resilience was something you built through effort and repetition, like training for a game.

But when chronic pain entered his life, his strategies stopped working. No matter how much he tried to push through, the pain didn't respond the way a sports injury would. It didn't follow the same rules. Frustrated, he started working with a therapist who specialized in chronic pain.

During their conversations, something unexpected surfaced. Andre found himself talking about his childhood in ways he never had before. His dad had been a hard man—strict, emotionally distant, and quick to criticize. Mistakes weren't tolerated. Weakness wasn't an option. Soccer had become Andre's refuge, the one place where he felt free, where he had a sense of control. He realized that his body had learned to hold tension early, not just from the game but from the unspoken pressure to never let his guard down.

For years, that drive had worked for him. He had become tough, reliable, able to push through anything. But now, his body wasn't cooperating, and he was beginning to see why. The same nervous system that had kept him sharp on the field had also kept him locked in high alert. Even long after leaving home, even after his playing days ended, that old tension was still there.

Andre wasn't broken. He had actually been resilient all along—just in ways he hadn't fully understood. Soccer had given him an outlet, a way to channel stress and structure his emotions, even before he had the words for it. Now, as he worked to heal his pain, he was realizing that resilience wasn't just about enduring. It was about learning when to soften, when to rest, and when to allow connection to do the work that sheer willpower couldn't.

His resilience had started as an internal skill. But moving forward, healing would also mean learning how to let others in.

It wasn't until Andre started working with a trauma-informed therapist that the pieces began to fall into place. He learned how his childhood experiences had shaped his nervous system, leaving it in a constant state of high alert. His body's overactive stress response had become a feedback loop, amplifying his pain.

THE HIDDEN LINKS BETWEEN TRAUMA AND CHRONIC PAIN

Trauma doesn't impact everyone in the same way. Here are some examples of how unresolved trauma might manifest as different kinds of chronic pain or related conditions:

- Migraines
- Chronic Back Pain
- Fibromyalgia
- Myalgic Encephalomyelitis/Chronic Fatigue Syndrome (ME/CFS)

These examples show how trauma can create lasting patterns in the body, even when the original experiences aren't consciously remembered. Understanding your own patterns is the first step toward healing.

Like Andre, many people don't recognize trauma in their lives because it doesn't fit the dramatic narratives they associate with the word. Trauma isn't just the result of catastrophic events; it can be any experience that overwhelms your nervous system's ability to cope, leaving lasting imprints on your body and mind.

Some trauma is acute, like an accident or assault. Other trauma is cumulative, built up over years—like growing up in a home where emotions weren't safe, where you felt unseen, or where you constantly had to prove your worth.

One framework for understanding trauma's long-term effects is **Adverse Childhood Experiences (ACEs)**—events such as:

- Physical, emotional, or sexual abuse
- Neglect, whether emotional or physical
- Growing up with a caregiver who struggled with addiction, mental illness, or violence

The ACEs study, a groundbreaking piece of research conducted by the Centers for Disease Control and Prevention (CDC) and Kaiser Permanente, revealed a startling connection: the more ACEs someone experienced, the higher their risk for chronic health problems, including chronic pain. Why? Because these early-life adversities shape the body's nervous, endocrine, and immune (NEI) systems, priming them to remain in a constant state of alarm.

For many people, trauma and chronic pain exist in a feedback loop. Unresolved trauma increases pain sensitivity, and persistent pain reinforces emotional distress. Over time, this cycle can become deeply ingrained in both the body and mind, making healing feel even more out of reach.

When you experience trauma, your body shifts into survival mode —what's often called fight, flight, or freeze. In the moment, this response helps you survive by preparing your body to escape or endure danger. But when trauma is chronic or unresolved, it disrupts your internal systems in ways that persist for decades.

For instance:

- Trauma can heighten your sensitivity to pain by keeping your body on high alert, even in safe situations.
- Stress hormones like cortisol can remain elevated or depleted, weakening your body's ability to heal.
- Inflammation caused by trauma can persist long after the event, amplifying chronic pain and fatigue.

SIDEBAR

Take Action: Exploring Your ACEs Score

The ACEs questionnaire helps you reflect on early-life experiences that may have contributed to your current challenges. While this exercise is not meant to diagnose or label, it can provide valuable insights into how your history might be influencing your health today.

Reflect on your experiences by answering the following questions in a yes or no fashion:

1. Did a parent or other adult in the household often swear at you, insult you, or humiliate you?
2. Did a parent or other adult in the household often push, grab, slap, or throw something at you?
3. Did you often feel that no one in your family loved you or thought you were important?
4. Did you often feel that you didn't have enough to eat, had to wear dirty clothes, or had no one to protect you?
5. Did you live with a household member who was depressed, mentally ill, or attempted suicide?
6. Did you live with someone who had a problem with alcohol or drugs?

7. Was your mother or stepmother often pushed, grabbed, slapped, or physically harmed?
8. Did your parents separate or divorce?
9. Were you ever sexually abused?
10. Was someone in your household incarcerated?

The ACEs questionnaire was developed as part of the Adverse Childhood Experiences (ACEs) study conducted by the Centers for Disease Control and Prevention (CDC) and Kaiser Permanente. For more information about the study and its findings, visitCDC ACEs Resource.

Step 1: Reflect on the types of adversities mentioned above.

- Count how many of these experiences apply to you.
- While your score doesn't define your future, it can help explain how early experiences shaped your body's stress responses and overall health.

Step 2: After identifying your score, consider journaling about how these experiences may connect to your current pain or stress patterns.

Step 3: Use this information to identify one area you'd like to focus on healing, such as stress management or emotional regulation.

INTEGRATING TRAUMA INTO THE PEAK RESILIENCE METHOD

Understanding how trauma affects the body underscores the importance of addressing all three pillars of the Peak Resilience Method—biological, psychological, and social resilience. By calming the nervous system, restoring balance to the endocrine system, and reducing inflammation in the immune system, you can begin to disrupt the trauma-pain cycle and create a foundation for healing.

First let's consider how trauma affects several of the bodily systems we talked about in Part One.

When trauma occurs, the body shifts into survival mode—fight, flight, or freeze. In the moment, this response is protective. But when trauma is unresolved or chronic, it disrupts your body's three key internal systems

1. The Nervous System – Overactive Alarm System

Your nervous system is designed to help you survive danger. When trauma occurs, your brain's amygdala, the alarm center, becomes hyperactive. It's constantly scanning for threats, even when there aren't any. At the same time, the prefrontal cortex, the rational part of your brain, loses its ability to regulate this alarm system. This leaves you stuck in a state of fight, flight, or freeze, unable to fully relax.

Over time, trauma strengthens neural pathways associated with fear and stress while weakening those associated with calm and resilience. This rewiring can make your nervous system hypersensitive, amplifying pain signals even in the absence of actual harm.

And it can lead to:

- Increased pain sensitivity
- Muscle tension and chronic stress responses
- Difficulty relaxing, even in safe environments

For Andre, this explained why his body was always tense, why relaxation felt so foreign, and why chronic pain had become so persistent. His body had learned to stay in a perpetual state of readiness, long after the original threat was gone.

2. The Endocrine System – The Stress Hormone Imbalance

The hypothalamic-pituitary-adrenal (HPA) axis is your body's stress management system. It connects your brain (the hypothalamus and pituitary gland) to your adrenal glands, which sit on top of your kidneys. Together, they release cortisol, a hormone that helps you respond to danger by increasing energy and focus.

Trauma disrupts this finely tuned system. Initially, cortisol levels may spike, keeping you in a constant state of readiness. But over time, the system can burn out, leading to low cortisol levels that leave you feeling exhausted and unable to recover properly. This dysregulation affects your sleep, energy, and ability to repair tissues—all of which are essential for managing chronic pain.

This creates two common patterns:

- Cortisol stays high → Leading to inflammation, poor sleep, and heightened pain
- Cortisol burns out (low levels) → Causing fatigue, immune dysfunction, and worsened pain regulation

Chronic pain sufferers often swing between these two states, which is why stress can make pain flare-ups so unpredictable.

3. The Immune System – Chronic Inflammation

Trauma activates the immune system's inflammatory response, flooding your body with chemicals like cytokines (e.g., interleukin-6 and tumor necrosis factor-alpha). These chemicals are helpful in the short term, helping you heal from injury or infection. But with unresolved trauma, the inflammatory response becomes chronic.

Chronic inflammation damages tissues, increases sensitivity to pain, and fuels neuroinflammation—irritation of the nervous system that amplifies the pain cycle. Even long after the traumatic event, your immune system may remain stuck in high alert, contributing to fatigue, pain, and other chronic health problems.

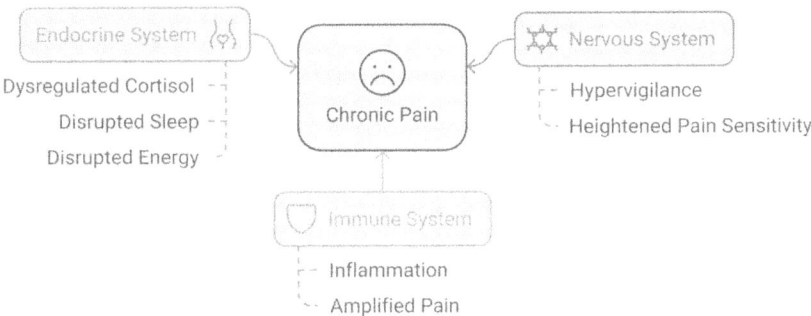

These disruptions to your internal systems are subtle and cumulative, which is why they can go unnoticed for years. But they're not permanent. By addressing trauma, you can begin to calm your nervous system, restore balance to your stress hormones, and reduce chronic inflammation, paving the way for healing.

SIDEBAR

Take Action: Checking In With the Body

Do you notice signs of trauma's effects in your body? For example, does your body feel tense, fatigued, or overly reactive to stress?

Which of the three systems—nervous, endocrine, or immune—feels most connected to your experience of pain?

After reflecting for a moment, move into these steps:

Step 1: Find a quiet space where you feel comfortable and safe. Sit or lie down in a relaxed position.

Step 2: Close your eyes (if that feels comfortable) and take a few deep breaths.

Step 3: Perform a body scan, slowly moving your attention from your head to your toes. Notice any areas of tension, discomfort, or numbness.

Step 4: Ask yourself:

- *Do certain parts of my body feel stuck in fight-or-flight mode?*
- *Do I notice tension that seems connected to a specific memory or emotion?*

Step 5: Write down your observations. What patterns do you notice?

BRIDGING INNER AND OUTER RESILIENCE

Not everyone who experiences trauma develops chronic pain. Why? Because resilience exists alongside trauma. Some people, like Andre, naturally develop coping mechanisms that help regulate their nervous system—even if they don't have the language for it.

Andre's experience with soccer had unknowingly helped him build psychological and biological resilience. The rhythmic movement, deep focus, and camaraderie of the game all helped regulate his nervous system. Without realizing it, his body was learning how to recover from stress in real-time.

This is key: resilience isn't just about avoiding pain—it's about what we do with it.

Even if someone develops inner resilience, pain can make it harder to connect with others. If trauma has taught you that people aren't safe, or if chronic pain has led to withdrawal from relationships, social resilience can suffer.

This is why healing isn't just an internal process—it's also a social process, the focus of our next two chapters.

For Andre, learning to name his trauma helped, but the real shift happened when he let himself trust others more. His therapist. His partner. Even an old teammate he hadn't reached out to in years. He was starting to understand that resilience wasn't just about facing things alone—it was about knowing when to lean on others.

Connection is not just emotional—it is biological. Social connection calms the nervous system, reduces cortisol, and helps the body regulate pain signals.

- Consider these questions:
- How has connection—or disconnection—played a role in your pain experience?
- Have you ever felt misunderstood or unseen in your pain?
- What relationships in your life feel safe? Which ones feel draining?
- How might social support influence your ability to heal?

Understanding the biological effects of trauma reinforces why healing requires a holistic approach. In the Peak Resilience Method, addressing trauma means working across all three pillars:

Biological Resilience: Calming the nervous system, balancing cortisol levels, and reducing inflammation.

Psychological Resilience: Rewiring thought patterns and emotions associated with trauma.

Social Resilience: Building relationships that create safety and trust, which are essential for recovery.

By addressing these interconnected systems, you can create a foundation for resilience that helps break the pain-trauma cycle. Later, in Part Four, we will begin looking in depth at trauma-specific methods for healing across the Peak Resilience Method.

Andre's emotional journey showed him that resilience wasn't about suppressing pain or toughing it out—it was about balance. He had spent his life building internal resilience without realizing it, but true healing required learning how to lean on others, too.

As we move into Part Four, we'll explore how relationships—whether with family, friends, or community—impact the way we experience pain. Because healing isn't just what happens inside us—it happens in the spaces between us, too.

CHAPTER-END AFFIRMATIONS

Reclaiming Strength, One Thought at a Time

Like many of us, and many of our patients, Andre never considered himself someone who had "trauma." But he did. And he was learning that healing wasn't about proving his strength. It was about allowing himself to soften in the right moments, to rest, to trust, and to connect.

These affirmations are meant to serve as reminders that trauma does not define you—your ability to heal does. Your nervous system, your body, and your mind are adaptable, and with each small step, you are moving toward greater balance, connection, and resilience.

- My past experiences have shaped me, but they do not have to control my future.
- I honor the ways my body has protected me, and I am learning new ways to feel safe.
- Healing is not about pushing through—it is about creating balance between strength and rest.
- I am allowed to soften. I am allowed to feel. I am allowed to heal.
- My nervous system can learn safety, and I am patient with the process.
- Connection is part of healing. I do not have to do this alone.
- The tension I hold is not my fault. I am learning how to release it, one breath at a time.
- I can rewrite the way my body and mind respond to stress, step by step.
- The patterns of the past do not define me—I am creating new ones.
- I am worthy of safety, of healing, and of relationships that support my resilience.

These words are not just reminders—they are the foundation for a new way of moving through the world, one that does not require carrying pain alone.

PART FOUR:
SOCIAL RESILIENCE – REWIRING CONNECTION

CHAPTER 9
THE SOCIAL COST OF CHRONIC PAIN

Raj had always been surrounded by people. His family's home was the center of gatherings, full of laughter, cousins running through the house, and meals that stretched late into the night. His friendships were just as strong—his college friends still messaged daily, checking in, planning weekend meetups. But after chronic pain entered his life, all of that changed.

At first, he tried to keep up. He pushed himself to attend family events, to smile through the pain. But each outing left him drained, sometimes bedridden for days. His body felt like a constant betrayal. When he began turning down invitations, the texts slowed. Eventually, they stopped.

Raj knew part of it was his own doing. In his cultural community, pain and illness were seen as something to endure privately. He had never known anyone to openly talk about chronic pain, and he wasn't about to be the first. When his mother would ask if he was feeling better, he nodded. When his friends joked about how he was always 'bailing,' he laughed along. He told himself it was easier this way.

But the loneliness became unbearable. He wasn't just losing people —he was losing himself.

Chronic pain doesn't just affect your body and your brain—it changes how you interact with the world. Pain can make it harder to show up for others, whether that means attending events, engaging in conversations, or simply having the emotional energy to connect. Over time, this can strain even the strongest relationships.

Loved ones may not understand what you're going through. Well-meaning friends might say things like, "Maybe you just need to get out more," or "You should try drinking more water," unknowingly invalidating your experience. Repeated misunderstandings create an invisible gap, making it feel easier to withdraw than to explain.

For Raj, the isolation wasn't just social—it felt deeply personal. He had always been the one people turned to, the friend who organized trips, the cousin who never missed a family gathering. Now, he didn't recognize himself. And worse, he didn't know how to ask for help.

FINDING CONNECTION AGAIN

Raj didn't set out to fix everything overnight. It started small.

First, he found a space where he felt understood. Late one night, unable to sleep, he searched for chronic pain support groups. He had no expectations but stumbled onto an online forum where people shared their stories, frustrations, and small victories. Reading their words felt like exhaling for the first time in months. Here, no one questioned his pain. No one told him to 'just push through.' They understood in a way even his closest friends could not.

For weeks, he just read posts. Then, one night, he wrote his own:

"I feel like I've disappeared. I used to be surrounded by friends and family, and now it feels like I don't exist. I don't even know how to explain this to them. Does anyone else feel this way?"

The responses came quickly. Some shared their own experiences, some offered words of encouragement, and a few suggested ways to talk to loved ones about chronic pain. One reply stood out:

"Start small. Connection doesn't have to mean long conversations or big gatherings. Even a text to someone you trust saying, 'I miss you,' is a step."

Raj wasn't sure he was ready for that. But it planted a seed.

Over the next few weeks, Raj took more small steps—commenting on a friend's post, sending a short voice message, responding to family group chats instead of leaving them unread. Each action reminded him that he wasn't as alone as he had feared.

THE EMOTIONAL TOLL OF ISOLATION

Living with chronic pain can lead to a sense of being trapped—not just in your body, but in your own mind. The emotional burden of feeling misunderstood or left out can create a cycle of withdrawal, where it feels safer to avoid others than risk being hurt or invalidated. This emotional isolation doesn't just feel bad; it also impacts your body.

Research shows that loneliness triggers the same stress responses as physical danger. When you feel disconnected, your brain's alarm system —the amygdala—becomes more active, increasing stress hormones like cortisol. Over time, this heightened stress can lead to inflammation and make pain feel more intense.

It's not just about other people misunderstanding you; chronic pain can change how you see yourself. You might worry about being a burden or feel frustrated that you can't contribute to relationships the way you used to. These feelings can create internal barriers to reaching out, making connection feel harder than ever.

But these barriers aren't permanent. Rebuilding connection starts with small, intentional actions, and the effort is worth it. Social resilience isn't about being perfect in your relationships—it's about finding ways to connect that feel meaningful and supportive for where you are right now.

SIDEBAR

Take Action: Finding Your Way Back

Think about a relationship that has changed since your pain began. What challenges have come up, and how have they affected you? What would rebuilding connection in that relationship look like?

Now try one or more of these steps today, another the next day, and another the day after:

- Reach out to one trusted person and share how you're feeling. Keep it simple, like saying, "I've been having a hard time and wanted to connect."
- Join an online or in-person support group to find people who understand your experiences.
- Practice gratitude by writing down one way someone has supported you, no matter how small.

THE SCIENCE OF SOCIAL RESILIENCE

Social connection is more than just a comfort—it's a biological necessity. Humans are wired to thrive in relationships, and when those connections are strong, they buffer the effects of stress, reduce inflammation, and promote healing. Conversely, loneliness and isolation take a toll on the body, amplifying pain and undermining resilience.

Understanding how social bonds influence the nervous, endocrine, and immune systems helps explain why connection is such a powerful tool for recovery.

When you feel connected to others, your brain releases *oxytocin*, often called the "bonding hormone." Oxytocin acts as a natural stress reliever, calming the amygdala—the brain's alarm center—and activating the parasympathetic nervous system, which shifts your body from "fight or flight" to "rest and repair." Oxytocin also helps regulate microglia, the immune cells in the brain responsible for controlling neuroinflammation. Studies by Dr. Sue Carter and others have demonstrated how oxytocin reduces the release of inflammatory cytokines like interleukin-6, which can heighten pain sensitivity.

Physical touch amplifies this effect. A simple hug, a pat on the shoulder, or holding hands can release *endorphins*, your body's natural painkillers. Endorphins interact with the *mu-opioid system* (covered last chapter), reducing pain perception and fostering a sense of safety and comfort. This is why even brief moments of connection can have an immediate calming effect, reducing feelings of fear and stress.

Loneliness, on the other hand, does the opposite. When social bonds weaken, the brain interprets isolation as a form of danger, keeping the amygdala on high alert. This chronic activation of the nervous system heightens pain sensitivity, creating a cycle where isolation feeds both physical and emotional distress.

Let's quickly look at how relationships, or the absence of relationship common in isolation, interact with several of the bodily systems from Part One.

The Endocrine System: Less Cortisol, More Balance

Supportive relationships also play a key role in regulating the hypothalamic-pituitary-adrenal (HPA) axis, the system that controls your stress response. When you feel connected and supported, your body releases less cortisol, the primary stress hormone.

This hormonal balance is essential for chronic pain recovery. High cortisol levels over time can disrupt sleep, increase inflammation, and make the body more sensitive to pain. By reducing cortisol, social connections give the body the breathing room it needs to focus on repair and recovery.

How Relationships Protect the Immune System

Loneliness and isolation don't just affect how you feel—they directly impact your immune system. People with strong social bonds tend to have lower levels of pro-inflammatory markers like interleukin-6 (IL-6) and tumor necrosis factor-alpha (TNF-α). These inflammatory molecules play a major role in neuroinflammation, which can amplify chronic pain and make the nervous system hypersensitive.

On the flip side, oxytocin—a hormone released during positive social interactions—has been shown to reduce these inflammatory markers. Oxytocin also helps regulate microglia, the immune cells in your brain that control neuroinflammation. When microglia are overactive, they make pain signals more intense. Calming them through social bonding reduces this sensitivity, creating a powerful biological pathway to healing.

The Ripple Effect of Connection

These systems—the nervous, endocrine, and immune—don't operate in isolation. Changes in one ripple out to the others, creating either positive or negative feedback loops.

Positive Feedback Loop of Connection

A supportive relationship calms the amygdala, reducing cortisol and inflammation. This makes it easier to manage pain and engage with others, reinforcing connection and resilience.

MASTERING CHRONIC PAIN

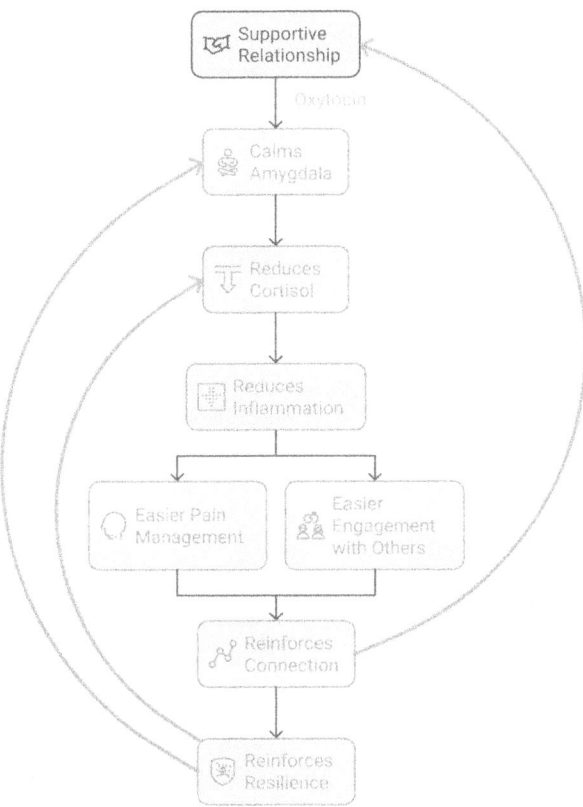

Negative Feedback Loop of Isolation

Loneliness triggers stress responses in the brain, increasing cortisol and inflammation. This makes pain worse, which can deepen feelings of isolation and withdrawal.

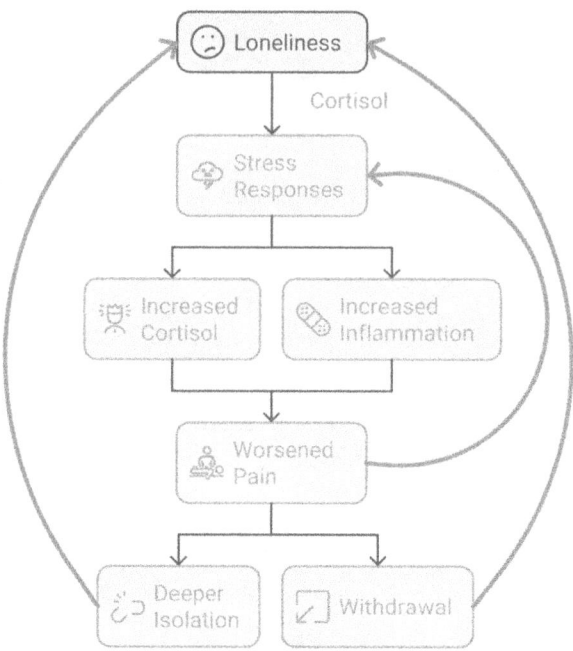

Breaking this cycle begins with small actions. Each moment of connection—whether it's a conversation, a hug, or simply feeling understood—activates your body's natural healing systems, turning the feedback loop in your favor.

EXPANDING SUPPORT: FINDING A COMMUNITY

Encouraged by the online group, Raj decided to take another step: attending an in-person chronic pain support group. It was easier knowing he wasn't going to be the only one navigating these challenges. At the first meeting, he listened more than he spoke. But as he heard others voice the same frustrations he had bottled up for so long, he felt something shift. He wasn't just a passive observer in his own life anymore—he was part of something again.

Later that evening, as he sat on the couch scrolling through posts from the group, his wife, Meera, walked in and sat beside him. She didn't say anything at first, just placed a warm hand on his knee.

"I saw you left early this morning," she finally said. "You never told me where you went."

Raj hesitated. For years, he had been hiding his pain from her, trying to carry it alone. He had told himself it was to protect her—to keep her from worrying, to hold on to some sense of dignity. But the truth was, he had been afraid. Afraid of looking weak. Afraid that if he let her in, he wouldn't be able to hold himself together.

But something was different now.

"I went to a support group," he admitted, his voice quieter than he expected. "For chronic pain."

Meera didn't look surprised. She nodded, her grip on his knee tightening slightly. "I'm glad," she said simply.

Raj let out a breath he hadn't realized he was holding. "You are?"

She turned to face him fully, searching his expression. "Raj, I've known something was wrong for a long time. I didn't push because I thought you needed to come to me when you were ready." She paused. "I've been waiting."

The weight of her words settled over him, heavy and warm at the same time. For so long, he had believed he was alone in this. That the pain was his to bear, that no one could truly understand what he was going through. But Meera had been there all along, waiting for him to let her in.

Raj swallowed hard. "I don't know how to talk about it," he admitted.

"You don't have to have the right words," she said. "Just don't shut me out."

That night, for the first time in years, Raj let himself lean into Meera's presence. He didn't try to smile through it. He didn't try to pretend. And when she simply held his hand in the quiet, he realized that connection didn't have to start big. It could begin with something as small as this.

REACHING OUT: SMALL STEPS TOWARD RECONNECTION

Over the next few weeks, Raj took more small steps—commenting on a friend's post, sending a short voice message, responding to family group chats instead of leaving them unread. It was Meera who encouraged him to open up to his family.

"They love you," she reminded him. "They just don't know what's happening. They can't help if you don't let them in."

Raj resisted at first, but eventually, he sent his sister a message:

"Hey. I know I've been distant. It's not because I don't care. I miss you."

The reply came almost immediately:

"I miss you too! Let's catch up soon?"

His heart thudded as he stared at the screen. It was such a simple response, but it meant more than he could explain.

The first time he spoke openly about his pain at a family dinner, his mother was quiet for a long time. Then she reached across the table, covering his hand with hers. "Beta, why didn't you tell us?" she asked softly.

Raj looked at his mother's face, at the worry etched into her expression, at his sister's furrowed brows and his father's steady gaze. "I didn't want to be a burden," he admitted.

His father shook his head. "Carrying this alone—that's the real burden, isn't it?"

It wasn't perfect. Some family members struggled to understand. Others asked too many questions or tried to offer quick-fix solutions. But overall, the relief of finally being seen outweighed the discomfort.

And that was enough for now.

HIDDEN PAIN: LIVING WITH AN INVISIBLE ILLNESS

Raj's pain didn't come from an accident, an injury, or anything that could be captured on a scan. There was no cast on his arm, no surgical scar to point to. His condition had a name—myalgic encephalomyelitis/chronic fatigue syndrome (ME/CFS)—but even saying it out loud often brought confusion or skepticism.

At first, even Raj had trouble believing it. Before ME/CFS, he had been active, social, and driven. He was a junior associate at a law firm. He played in a tennis league. He swam regularly at his local YMCA. He had prided himself on his ability to push through exhaustion, to work hard, to be the person others could rely on. But then the fatigue started creeping in—not the kind that a nap could fix, but a crushing exhaustion that made it feel like his muscles were made of lead.

Then came the brain fog. Words slipped from his mind mid-sentence, emails took twice as long to compose, and once-effortless tasks felt insurmountable. He felt feverish without a fever, sore without injury, wiped out after something as simple as a short walk or conversation.

Doctors ran tests, but they all came back normal. Some told him he was stressed. Others suggested he was just out of shape (which he found laughable considering how active he was) that he needed to "push through." One even asked if he was depressed. But Raj wasn't sad—he was frustrated, desperate for someone to see that something was wrong.

Finally, after months of bouncing between specialists, a neurologist gave him the diagnosis: ME/CFS. But even then, the relief of having a name was quickly overshadowed by something else—the realization that many people, even in the medical field, didn't believe his illness was real.

THE STIGMA OF CHRONIC ILLNESS

Unlike a visible injury or a well-known disease, conditions like ME/CFS and fibromyalgia exist in a frustrating space where symptoms are debilitating, but proof is elusive. There are no clear biomarkers, no definitive tests that a doctor can point to and say, "Here it is." Instead, patients are often left navigating a world that expects tangible evidence before offering validation.

For Raj, this meant encountering reactions that ranged from doubt to outright dismissal. His employer was initially sympathetic, but as his sick days accumulated, the patience wore thin. "You don't look sick," his boss said more than once. And the unspoken message beneath it was clear: *So why can't you just push through?*

Even within his family, the responses were mixed. His mother was worried but confused. "You're young and strong," she said. "Maybe you just need to rest more." His father, ever pragmatic, suggested *more* exercise. His friends, who once called him reliable, started calling him unreliable. The more he struggled to keep up, the more invitations stopped coming.

The isolation didn't just stem from the pain itself, but from the constant need to prove that it existed.

How Society Misunderstands Conditions Like ME/CFS and Fibromyalgia

For those living with chronic pain conditions that lack clear medical markers, the barriers to understanding are deeply ingrained. There are several reasons why illnesses like ME/CFS and fibromyalgia remain so stigmatized and misunderstood:

- They don't show up on standard tests. Unlike a broken bone or a torn ligament, these conditions don't have definitive imaging or blood tests that prove their existence. This often leads to misdiagnosis, skepticism, or outright dismissal—especially from medical professionals who rely on objective data to guide treatment.
- Symptoms are inconsistent. On some days, Raj could function almost normally. On others, he could barely get out of bed. This unpredictability confused those around him. "But you were fine yesterday," people would say, as though that invalidated what he was feeling today.
- The fatigue isn't "just being tired." People often compared his exhaustion to how they felt after a long workday or a bad night's sleep. But ME/CFS fatigue isn't ordinary tiredness—it's post-exertional malaise, where even minor

exertion can trigger a full-body crash that lasts for days or weeks.
- Pain is subjective, making it easier to dismiss. Chronic pain isn't visible, and because it varies from person to person, it's often downplayed as exaggerated or psychological. The phrase "it's all in your head" is something nearly every ME/CFS and fibromyalgia patient has heard at least once.
- Cultural stigma around weakness and endurance. In many communities, including Raj's, there is an unspoken expectation to endure suffering silently. Pain is something to be pushed through, not something to shape your identity around. This made it even harder for Raj to admit when he needed help.

The weight of these misunderstandings made Raj's isolation worse. He wasn't just fighting his body—he was fighting a world that didn't believe him.

Breaking the Cycle: Acknowledging Hidden Pain

The turning point came when Raj finally allowed himself to name what he was experiencing—not just to himself, but to those around him.

At his chronic pain support group, he met others with fibromyalgia, ME/CFS, post-viral syndromes, and other invisible illnesses. They, too, had heard the doubts, had faced the skepticism, had spent years second-guessing themselves.

"You don't need anyone's permission to believe your own pain," one of them told him. And that sentence, more than anything, helped Raj begin to reclaim his story.

Instead of exhausting himself trying to convince people who wouldn't listen, he started focusing on those who did. His wife, Meera, had been waiting for him to let her in. His sister, who had initially struggled to understand, started checking in more often, asking, *"How are you feeling today?"* instead of *"Are you better yet?"* His support group gave him language for what he was going through, a space where he didn't have to prove anything.

And most importantly, he stopped doubting and criticizing himself.

Yes, his condition was real. Yes, his pain was real. And yes, he deserved to be believed, even if the world didn't always make space for that truth.

Raj's story is a reminder that while chronic pain isolates, connection heals. Small, intentional steps toward reconnection—whether with a support group, a trusted friend, or even yourself—can shift the cycle from isolation to resilience.

CHAPTER-END RESOURCE

Checklist for Acts of Connection

1. Send a text
2. Share a hug
3. Join a support group
4. Write a short thank you note to someone who has supported you
5. Volunteer for a cause that you care about
6. Create a shared project, like planting a garden
7. Invite someone for a cup of coffee
8. Say "Thank you" to someone in your daily routine

CHAPTER-END ACTIVITY

A Step Towards Reconnection

Think of a time when a conversation or interaction left you feeling calmer or supported. How did it affect your mood, pain levels, or stress?

Now, consider:

- What's one small action you could take this week to strengthen a relationship or create a new connection?
- Who in your life could benefit from a moment of intentional connection?

Pick one person in your life to reach out to this week. It could be as simple as sending a text, making a phone call, or asking to meet for coffee. Focus on being present in the moment rather than striving for a "perfect" interaction.

If you need to start smaller, how about a letter?

Write a letter to someone you'd like to reconnect with. You don't have to send it right away—or at all—but use it as an opportunity to express your feelings, share your experience, and outline what rebuilding trust might look like.

CHAPTER 10
CULTIVATING SOCIAL RESILIENCE

Social connection is more than just a comfort—it's a biological necessity. Humans are wired to thrive in relationships, and strong connections can buffer the effects of stress, reduce inflammation, and promote healing. When we lose those connections, the body and mind don't just suffer emotionally—they enter a heightened state of distress, which has real, measurable consequences.

When you feel connected, your brain releases oxytocin, a hormone that acts as a natural stress reliever. Oxytocin dampens the brain's alarm center—the amygdala—helping to reduce fear and anxiety. This shift moves the nervous system out of "fight or flight" mode and into "rest and repair" mode, allowing the body to focus on healing rather than stress.

Physical touch—like a hug, holding hands, or even a reassuring hand on the shoulder—can trigger the release of endorphins, the body's natural painkillers. These interactions signal safety and comfort to the brain, reducing pain perception and promoting a sense of well-being.

Even brief moments of social engagement—talking to a friend, sharing a laugh, or feeling understood—activate the ventral Vagus nerve, part of the parasympathetic nervous system that promotes calm and relaxation. When this system is engaged, inflammation decreases, stress hormones stabilize, and the body can recover more efficiently.

THE IMPACT OF ISOLATION: WHEN LONELINESS BECOMES PAIN

Loneliness, on the other hand, does the opposite. Studies show that social isolation triggers the brain's stress response, increasing cortisol levels, raising inflammation, and amplifying pain perception. Over time, this creates a destructive cycle: pain leads to isolation, isolation increases stress, and stress worsens pain.

One of the most well-known studies on the biological effects of loneliness comes from psychologist John Cacioppo, whose research demonstrated that chronic loneliness increases the activity of genes involved in inflammation. His work found that socially isolated individuals had heightened levels of pro-inflammatory cytokines, which contribute to chronic pain and disease. This inflammatory response mimics what happens during physical illness or injury, suggesting that the body treats loneliness as a kind of biological threat.

A groundbreaking experiment by neuroscientist Eisenberger and Lieberman at UCLA showed that social rejection activates the same brain regions as physical pain—specifically, the anterior cingulate cortex (ACC), which is involved in processing both emotional and physical distress. In the study, participants played a virtual ball-tossing game, believing they were interacting with real people. When they were excluded from the game, fMRI scans showed their brains reacted as if they had experienced physical harm. This demonstrated that the pain of loneliness is not metaphorical—the brain processes it in the same way it processes bodily pain.

The pain of isolation isn't just emotional; it has real, physiological consequences:

- **Chronic stress response** – Persistent loneliness keeps the body in a low-grade fight-or-flight state, increasing cortisol and inflammation.

- **Heightened pain sensitivity** – The brain becomes more sensitive to pain signals, making even minor discomfort feel overwhelming.
- **Disrupted sleep cycles** – Loneliness increases nighttime cortisol levels, making restful sleep more difficult and increasing fatigue-related pain.
- **Weakened immune function** – Long-term social isolation suppresses immune responses, making the body more vulnerable to illness and slower to heal.

Studies on people with chronic pain conditions like fibromyalgia have found that social support is one of the strongest predictors of pain levels. Those with strong, supportive relationships reported lower pain intensity, fewer flare-ups, and better emotional resilience, while those who felt isolated experienced worse symptoms.

WHY SOME FORMS OF ISOLATION FEEL WORSE THAN OTHERS

Not all isolation is the same. Research has shown that perceived isolation—the feeling that no one understands you—is even more damaging than being physically alone. Someone can be surrounded by people but still feel emotionally isolated if they don't feel seen or heard.

As established last chapter, for individuals with conditions like fibromyalgia, myalgic encephalomyelitis/chronic fatigue syndrome (ME/CFS), or persistent post-injury pain, this can be even more pronounced. Unlike a visible injury (such as a broken bone or post-surgical pain), these conditions don't have obvious external markers. Many people with these conditions face skepticism, dismissal, or frustration from others, making them feel even more alone.

Raj had experienced this firsthand. He often felt that if he had a cast on his leg, or some kind of visible injury, people would understand his pain. But his condition was invisible, and that invisibility made the isolation feel worse. When he told people about his chronic pain, he could see the skepticism in their eyes—the doubt, the assumption that he was exaggerating. Over time, he stopped trying to explain. He just withdrew.

Breaking the Cycle: Connection as Medicine

If social isolation feeds pain, then social connection can be part of the solution. Studies have found that simple acts of meaningful connection—whether through family, friends, or support groups—can have measurable effects on pain reduction.

A study published in the Journal of Pain found that patients who engaged in regular social interactions reported lower pain levels than those who remained isolated.

Harvard's famous "Longevity Study" found that the single biggest predictor of long-term health and well-being wasn't diet or exercise—it was the strength of one's social relationships.

Research on cancer patients has shown that those with strong social support networks have better treatment outcomes, lower levels of pain, and longer survival rates.

For Raj, the science of isolation helped him understand what he had been experiencing. His pain wasn't just in his body—it was being amplified by loneliness, by the stress of disconnection. If isolation was worsening his pain, then maybe connection—real, intentional connection—could help ease it.

That realization didn't make reaching out easier overnight. But it gave him a reason to try.

SOCIAL RESILIENCE AND THE PEAK RESILIENCE METHOD

Raj wasn't sure how long he had been standing in the doorway. Long enough for the tea in his mug to cool, long enough to hear his wife Meera's voice float down the hall as she laughed at something on the phone. For a long time, that sound had been background noise, something he had barely registered. But tonight, it was a reminder of the space between them.

He had spent so much time pulling away—from her, from his friends, from the world outside their home—that returning felt impossible. Every time Meera asked how he was feeling, he gave the same answer: "I'm fine." Even though he wasn't.

Reaching out had seemed impossible at first. Where would he even start? But his support group had given him something he hadn't realized he needed: proof that he wasn't alone.

"Start small," one of them had said. "Connection isn't about fixing everything at once—it's about choosing to step toward someone, even if it's just an inch."

Maybe that was what social resilience really was—not about having flawless relationships, but about choosing to stay in them, even when pain made him want to disappear.

Social resilience isn't just about feeling connected—it's a biological force that impacts every area of your well-being. When you foster meaningful relationships, you activate pathways in your brain that calm the nervous system, balance stress hormones, and reduce inflammation. These changes don't just help you feel better in the moment; they create the conditions for long-term healing.

In the Peak Resilience Method, social resilience is one of the three foundational pillars, alongside biological and psychological resilience. It strengthens your ability to manage stress, regulate emotions, and heal from the inside out. Social resilience also amplifies the effects of other practices. For instance:

- Mindfulness is more effective when practiced in a supportive environment.
- Healthy habits like exercise or nutrition are easier to sustain with encouragement from loved ones.
- Emotional healing accelerates when you feel seen and understood by others.

For Raj, understanding this was one thing. Living it was another. He had always thought of resilience as something personal, something built alone. But isolation had only made him feel weaker, not stronger. Maybe healing wasn't just about what he could endure alone, but about who he could endure it with.

WHY TRUST IS ESSENTIAL FOR CONNECTION

Raj hesitated before opening the door to the living room. Meera was still on the phone, but when she noticed him, her face softened. "I'll call you back," she said into the receiver, setting it aside.

"You okay?" she asked.

Raj wanted to say yes. But something inside him stopped. He had spent months pretending everything was fine. And where had that gotten him? Alone.

"I… don't know how to do this," he admitted, running a hand through his hair. "Talking about it. Explaining. I don't even know where to start."

Meera's face didn't shift with impatience. She didn't push. She just waited.

"You don't have to have the perfect words," she said after a moment. "Just don't shut me out."

Raj exhaled. The truth was chronic pain had made him doubt everything about himself. He worried he was a burden. That he wasn't the same person Meera had married. That his exhaustion, his cancellations, his lack of energy had taken something from them both.

For many people living with chronic pain, these fears create internal barriers to connection. You might:

- Worry about being a burden to the people you love.
- Feel frustrated that you can't contribute as much as before.
- Experience resentment when others don't seem to understand.

These emotions are valid—but they can also become walls. Rebuilding trust starts by addressing these challenges, both within yourself and in your relationships.

Trust is the foundation of every meaningful relationship, but chronic pain can challenge that foundation. Friends and family members may not fully understand what you're going through, and their well-meaning advice can feel dismissive or even hurtful. Repeated misunderstandings—like suggestions to "just relax" or "Maybe you just need to think more positively"—can leave you feeling unseen, creating emotional distance.

At the same time, living with pain can make you more self-critical in relationships. You might worry about being a burden or feel frustrated that you can't contribute as much as you used to. These fears can lead to withdrawal, which deepens feelings of isolation.

Rebuilding trust starts by addressing these challenges—both the misunderstandings with others and the self-doubt within yourself. By creating space for honest communication and small steps toward connection, you can begin to restore the bonds that chronic pain may have strained.

HOW TO REBUILD TRUST AND STRENGTHEN RELATIONSHIPS

1. Open Communication

Start by sharing your experience with honesty and vulnerability. This doesn't mean you have to share every detail of your pain, but letting loved ones know how it affects your energy, emotions, and availability can help them understand your needs. For example:

- "Sometimes the pain leaves me exhausted, and I might need to rest instead of making plans. It doesn't mean I don't care about spending time with you."

Use "I" statements to express your feelings and needs without placing blame:

- "I feel overwhelmed when I get suggestions for treatments I've already tried. What I need most is someone to listen and be there for me."

2. Set Clear Boundaries

Protecting your energy is vital when living with chronic pain. Boundaries allow you to say no to activities or conversations that drain you while staying connected in ways that feel sustainable. For instance:

- If a family gathering feels too overwhelming, offer an alternative: "I can't make it to dinner, but I'd love to catch up with you for a coffee next week."

3. Acknowledge Past Tensions

If chronic pain has caused misunderstandings or distance in a relationship, addressing those tensions openly can help rebuild trust. You might say:

- "I know I've pulled back a lot lately, and I'm sorry if that's hurt you. I've been trying to manage the pain and figure out how to balance everything. I'd like to reconnect and find ways to support each other."

4. Focus on Small Moments of Connection

Trust isn't rebuilt overnight. Small, consistent actions—like responding to a text, sharing a laugh, or showing appreciation—lay the groundwork for deeper bonds. Celebrate these moments as wins, even if they seem minor.

5. Seek Understanding Together

Consider inviting loved ones to learn more about chronic pain with you. Sharing resources or attending a support group together can help them better understand your experience and how to support you.

SIDEBAR

Take Action: Relationship Check-In

How do your relationships support—or challenge—your resilience? What's one step you could take to strengthen a connection that uplifts you?

Think about a relationship you'd like to rebuild. What specific steps could you take to foster trust and understanding in that relationship?

As you explore these strategies, remember that building connection takes time and patience. Each small act, whether it's reaching out to a loved one or joining a community group, is a step toward greater resilience. These efforts don't just improve your social life—they create the conditions for healing and thriving.

And remember that not every relationship can—or should—be rebuilt. If someone consistently invalidates your experience or disregards your boundaries, it may be healthier to step back or let go. This doesn't mean you've failed; it means you're prioritizing relationships that uplift and support you.

Understanding how social connection affects your body highlights its importance, but knowledge alone isn't enough. The next step is turning these insights into action, using simple strategies to build and strengthen meaningful relationships.

SIDEBAR

Take Action: Building Your Social Resilience Plan

1. **Identify Your Circles of Support**

Write down the names of people, groups, or communities you feel connected to—or would like to connect with.

2. **Set Small Goals for Connection**

For each name or group, write down one action you can take this month to strengthen that relationship. Examples might include:

- Sending a text or email.
- Scheduling a short phone call.
- Attending a meeting or event.

3. **Reflect on Your Progress**

At the end of the month, revisit your list. Which actions felt the most meaningful? How did they impact your sense of connection and resilience?

PRACTICAL STEPS TO BUILD SOCIAL RESILIENCE

Building social resilience doesn't require grand gestures or dramatic changes. It's about taking small, intentional steps that feel manageable, especially when energy and pain levels vary day to day. These steps can help you reconnect with others, find new sources of support, and foster a sense of belonging.

1. Start with Small Acts to Rebuild Connection

Rebuilding connection begins with small, intentional steps. Chronic pain can make relationships feel distant or strained, but even brief moments of outreach can create a ripple effect. These acts don't have to be elaborate—they're about showing care and creating opportunities for trust and closeness to grow.

Here are some simple ways to reconnect:

- **Send a Message**

A short text or email can remind someone you're thinking of them. For example: *"Hi, I've been thinking about you and hope you're doing well. Let's catch up soon!"*

- **Compliment or Thank Someone**

Kind words can brighten someone's day while strengthening your bond. Consider writing a quick thank-you note or sharing a compliment.

- **Share a Small Moment**

Reconnect over shared interests, like watching a favorite movie, solving a puzzle, or discussing a book. These low-energy activities foster connection without the need for deep conversations.

- **Practice Kindness**

Offering help with a task, expressing appreciation, or simply listening to someone can deepen relationships while boosting your own resilience.

- **Attend a Group or Class**

  Join a support group or participate in a shared-interest activity to meet new people who understand your challenges or share your passions.

Each small act builds a foundation for deeper relationships. Focus on what feels manageable for you and let connection grow at its own pace.

2. **Rebuild Relationships Gently**

If chronic pain has caused distance or misunderstandings in certain relationships, rebuilding trust is possible—but it often starts small. Begin by expressing appreciation or acknowledging past tensions with honesty. For example:

- "I've missed spending time with you, but my energy has been limited lately. I'd like to find ways to reconnect."
- "I know I've been distant while managing my pain, and I appreciate your patience."

Rebuilding doesn't have to happen all at once. Focus on small moments of reconnection, like a quick phone call or a short visit, and let trust grow naturally.

While rebuilding individual relationships is crucial, community connection offers a broader network of support. Finding people who understand your challenges or share your passions can deepen your resilience in ways that complement personal relationships.

3. Find Community Support

Connecting with others who share your experiences can be profoundly validating. Support groups, shared-interest clubs, or online communities provide opportunities to bond over common challenges and passions.

- Look for local or virtual support groups for people living with chronic pain.
- Join a class or club related to a hobby you enjoy, like gardening, painting, or book discussions.
- Explore volunteer opportunities, which can foster connection while giving you a sense of purpose.

For many, online communities offer a unique advantage: they provide connection from the comfort of home, making it easier to engage even on days when pain or energy levels make in-person meetings difficult. These spaces often bring together people from diverse backgrounds, allowing for a wide range of shared experiences and advice.

However, not all online communities are created equal. Some groups can unintentionally become places where negativity, unhelpful comparisons, or misinformation thrive. Take care when choosing where to engage. Look for communities that focus on empowerment, evidence-based information, and fostering resilience. Search for online support groups focused on chronic pain or resilience. When exploring a group, notice how the tone of conversations makes you feel. Does the group leave you feeling more hopeful and supported? If not, it might be worth seeking a different space.

4. Focus on Physical Connection

Physical touch is one of the most powerful ways to release oxytocin, often called the "bonding hormone." Oxytocin calms your nervous system, reduces stress, and creates a sense of safety and comfort. Simple gestures like a hug, holding hands, or sitting close to someone you trust can have profound effects, especially during times of stress or pain.

However, physical connection isn't always accessible or comfortable for everyone. If you've experienced trauma or find physical touch overwhelming, there are still ways to nurture connection and calm through self-soothing practices. These techniques allow you to foster resilience in a way that feels safe and empowering.

Havening Touch

Havening Touch is a gentle, trauma-informed practice developed by Dr. Ronald Ruden and Dr. Steven Ruden. It involves self-administered physical motions to create a sense of safety and calm. By lightly stroking your arms, hands, or face in soothing motions, you can activate your parasympathetic nervous system—the body's natural "rest and repair" mode.

How to Practice Havening Touch:

- Cross your arms and gently stroke from your shoulders down to your elbows, repeating this motion slowly and rhythmically.
- Alternatively, place your hands on your cheeks and lightly stroke downward toward your jawline.
- As you practice, focus on a calming phrase, such as *"I am safe now,"* or visualize a peaceful scene, like a beach or forest.

Havening Touch has been shown to help individuals reduce stress, ease trauma responses, and foster resilience by soothing the brain's alarm system. This technique provides a sense of control and safety, making it particularly beneficial for those navigating trauma or chronic pain. To learn more about Havening, visit www.havening.org.

Tapping (Emotional Freedom Techniques)

Tapping, also known as Emotional Freedom Techniques (EFT), was developed by **Gary Craig** as a way to combine principles of traditional Chinese acupressure with modern psychology. It involves gently tapping specific points on the body, such as the forehead, collarbone, or chest, while focusing on calming thoughts or emotions.

How to Practice Tapping:

- Identify a specific area of discomfort or emotion (e.g., anxiety, fear, or pain).
- Use your fingertips to tap lightly on key points, such as the side of your hand, the space above your eyebrows, or the top of your chest.
- Repeat a calming statement, such as *"Even though I feel this pain, I am working toward peace."*

Research has shown that EFT can help reduce stress, manage pain, and improve emotional well-being by calming the nervous system and balancing energy pathways in the body. For more information on EFT, visit www.emofree.com.

Time with Pets

If physical touch with others isn't an option, spending time with a pet can have similar calming effects. Stroking a dog's fur, cuddling with a cat, or even watching fish swim in an aquarium releases oxytocin and lowers stress levels. Pets provide non-judgmental companionship, helping to ease feelings of loneliness and isolation.

Self-Compassionate Gestures

Sometimes, simple gestures of self-compassion can create a sense of safety and comfort:

- Place a hand on your heart and take slow, deep breaths.
- Rub your hands together to create warmth, then hold them gently against your face or chest.
- Sit in a comfortable position, close your eyes, and gently rock back and forth.

These gestures can help calm your nervous system and remind you that you're not alone in your experience.

The Power of Physical Connection

Whether it's through a hug from a loved one, a moment of self-soothing, or time with a pet, physical connection—external or internal—plays a vital role in building resilience. These practices reduce stress, calm the nervous system, and create a foundation for healing.

Experiment with the techniques that feel most accessible and meaningful to you and remember that even small moments of connection can have a profound impact on your body and mind.

5. **Practice Acts of Kindness**

Engaging in acts of kindness benefits both the giver and the receiver, boosting oxytocin and strengthening social bonds. These can be as simple as:

- Offering to help someone with a small task.
- Complimenting a stranger or coworker.

- Writing a thank-you note to someone who has supported you.

Kindness doesn't just help others—it reinforces your own sense of connection and purpose.

6. Set Boundaries for Healthy Relationships

Not every relationship is beneficial to your resilience. Setting clear boundaries allows you to protect your energy and prioritize connections that uplift and support you. For example:

- Politely declining invitations that feel overwhelming: "I appreciate the invite, but I'll need to rest that day. Let's plan something quieter soon."
- Limiting conversations about treatments or advice that feel unhelpful: "Thank you for your concern, but I'd rather focus on other topics right now."

Healthy boundaries create space for relationships to thrive on mutual respect and understanding.

Which of these steps feels most approachable for you to try this week? How might it strengthen your sense of connection?

SIDEBAR

Take Action: *Connection Map*

Take a blank piece of paper and draw a circle in the center with your name in it. Around the circle, write the names of people or communities you feel connected to—or would like to reconnect with. Reflect on one action you can take for each connection this week, whether it's sending a message, expressing gratitude, or planning a conversation.

THE HEALING POWER OF CONNECTION

Chronic pain can make the world feel smaller, isolating you from the people and experiences that once brought joy and meaning to your life. When every interaction feels like effort and every explanation feels like an uphill battle, withdrawing can seem like the easier choice. But pain thrives in isolation, and disconnection feeds the cycle of stress, inflammation, and suffering.

Connection, however—whether through a supportive friend, a shared moment of kindness, or a newfound community—has the power to break that cycle. When you begin to reach out, even in small ways, you send a signal to your body that you are not alone, that you are safe, that you belong.

Raj never thought a simple text message to his sister would change anything. He had spent so long convincing himself that he was better off handling things alone, that no one would understand, that it was too exhausting to explain. But that first message, the simple I miss you, chipped away at the distance he had created. His family hadn't given up on him; they had just been waiting for him to let them back in.

The science is clear: relationships aren't just emotional support—they are biological allies. They calm your nervous system, reduce inflammation, and buffer stress, creating a physical environment in which healing becomes possible. A simple hug, a shared laugh, or the warmth of someone who listens without judgment can activate powerful healing mechanisms within your brain and body.

But connection isn't just about reducing pain. It's about reclaiming yourself.

Imagine what's possible if you begin to nurture those connections today. What might it feel like to rebuild trust, to find understanding, to rediscover a sense of belonging? What if connection didn't have to feel like an obligation—but instead, like a lifeline pulling you back toward the world?

Every small step you take toward connection strengthens your resilience. With each act of kindness, each moment of outreach, and each shared experience, you are laying the foundation for a life that feels fuller, richer, and more meaningful.

CHAPTER-END ACTIVITY

Reconnecting and Building Resilience

Reconnection doesn't have to be a grand gesture—it begins with small, intentional actions. Chronic pain can make relationships feel distant or strained, but every small step you take strengthens the foundation of trust, understanding, and support.

Use this activity to reflect on your relationships and create an actionable plan to nurture them.

Step 1: Focus on Quality, Not Quantity
Connection isn't about how many people you interact with—it's about the depth and meaning of those interactions.

Reflect:
Who in your life makes you feel safe and supported?
Are there relationships that drain your energy rather than uplift you?
How can you prioritize spending time with those who encourage and support you?

Actionable Step:
Choose one person this week to connect with more intentionally—whether through a conversation, a message, or simply sharing a moment together.

Step 2: Rebuild Relationships Gently
If pain has created distance in a relationship, rebuilding trust takes time. It's okay to start small.

Reflect:
Has a specific relationship changed since your pain began?

What emotions come up when you think about reconnecting?
What would rebuilding trust look like in a way that feels safe for you?

Actionable Step:
Choose one phrase you can use to open the door to reconnection, such as: *"I've missed spending time with you. I'd love to reconnect." "I know I've been distant, and I appreciate your patience. Let's find a way to connect that works for both of us."*

Step 3: Explore New Connections
Sometimes, meaningful connection comes from outside of your existing circle. Expanding your support system can provide validation, encouragement, and fresh perspectives.

Reflect:
Where could you find people who share your experiences or interests? What type of community would feel supportive and uplifting for you?

Actionable Step:
Explore one of the following options:

- Join a local or online chronic pain support group.
- Sign up for an interest-based activity (art, gardening, book clubs).
- Volunteer for a cause you care about to foster new connections.

Step 4: Set Boundaries While Reconnecting
Rebuilding relationships doesn't mean overextending yourself. It's okay to communicate your limits while still prioritizing connection.

Reflect:
What personal boundaries do you need to protect your energy? How can you communicate your needs in a way that maintains connection?

Actionable Step:
Choose one boundary statement to use this week:

- "I'd love to join, but I'll need to keep it short today to conserve my energy."
- "I appreciate your concern, but I'd rather focus on how we can reconnect rather than discussing my health challenges."

Connection doesn't have to happen all at once. Each small step creates a ripple effect—strengthening your resilience and rebuilding the relationships that matter most.

CHAPTER-END AFFIRMATIONS

Social Resilience and You

Take a deep breath and remind yourself: Connection is healing. It is not about perfection—it is about showing up, one small step at a time. Let these affirmations guide and support you as you strengthen your social resilience.

Affirmations for Trusting in Connection:

- I am worthy of love, support, and understanding.
- My pain does not make me a burden; I am still whole and valuable.
- I choose to believe that I am not alone in this journey.
- I allow myself to be seen and heard by those who care about me.

Affirmations for Rebuilding Relationships:

- Small steps toward connection are meaningful and enough.
- I give myself permission to set boundaries while still fostering connection.
- It is safe for me to reach out and ask for what I need.
- My relationships can grow and change in ways that support my well-being.

Affirmations for Healing Through Community:

- I am open to finding people who understand and uplift me.
- I deserve relationships that bring me comfort, not stress.
- By nurturing connections, I create space for my body and mind to heal.
- I embrace the strength that comes from being part of a supportive community.

Affirmations for Letting Go of Isolation:

- Even when I feel alone, I remind myself that connection is still possible.
- My pain does not define me or isolate me—I choose to step toward connection.
- I replace self-doubt with self-compassion as I rebuild trust in relationships.
- Every small act of connection is a victory, a step toward resilience.

PART FIVE:
YOUR RESILIENCE CODE

Throughout the first several parts of the book we've taken a journey to better understand how pain affects us across biological, psychological, and social spectrums. We've met several patients who, just like you, have watched their world's become increasingly narrow due to pain, only to discover that resiliency is the path towards empowerment. We've covered a variety of exercises and tips for beginning to build resiliency across the biopsychosocial model.

Now, in our final chapters, it's time to tie everything together and embark on building your own personal framework, what we call the Peak Resilience Method. In the following chapters we'll talk about the role of amplifiers; revisit healing from trauma; move through specific activities and plans for developing biological resilience, psychological resilience, and social resilience; consider the importance of mindset for continued success; then end with your personalized Resilience Code under the Peak Resilience Method.

Think of this final part of the book as a personal guide that you can carry forward in your journey of taking your life back from chronic pain.

A QUICK NOTE ABOUT SAFETY

The strategies in these practical chapters are designed to support your resilience across the biopsychosocial model. But please remember: **this book is not a substitute for medical advice**, and reading it does **not establish a doctor–patient relationship** with any of the authors.

Everyone's body is different. What works well for one person may not work—or may even cause harm—for another. This is especially true when it comes to medications or supplements, which can interact with existing conditions or prescriptions. **If you're considering adding or adjusting any treatment, medication, or supplement, please consult with your healthcare provider first.** They can help you evaluate what's safe, effective, and appropriate for your individual needs.

We've made every effort to provide well-researched, evidence-informed suggestions in these chapters, but they are meant as general guidance—not specific instructions. Your safety, context, and care plan should always come first.

CHAPTER 11
THE POWER OF AMPLIFIERS

Chronic pain often feels like a storm that refuses to pass, overwhelming every aspect of life. At its core, the persistence of this pain is tied to amplifiers—biological, psychological, and social forces that magnify dysfunction and sustain the pain cycle. These amplifiers don't operate in isolation; they interact with one another, creating self-reinforcing feedback loops that intensify the experience of pain.

Imagine the screech of a microphone placed too close to a speaker. The sound feeds back on itself, growing louder and more unbearable. Amplifiers in chronic pain function in much the same way. For instance, stress heightens the body's sensitivity to pain, while the pain itself creates more stress. Similarly, the isolation often caused by chronic pain erodes emotional support, deepening feelings of distress and hopelessness. These loops work in tandem, making it feel as though the pain is controlling every part of life.

Understanding this process is key to breaking the cycle. Each amplifier holds the potential to either sustain pain or, when addressed, to amplify healing and resilience. By identifying and disrupting these feedback loops, you can begin to reverse their effects and reclaim control.

Chronic pain is sustained through interconnected loops: biologically, pain triggers inflammation, which further sensitizes the nervous system, heightening pain perception. Psychologically, the fear of pain often leads to avoidance, which increases tension and anxiety, feeding back into the pain cycle. Socially, isolation—whether physical or emotional—reduces the support needed to cope, leaving you feeling more alone and overwhelmed. These loops are not separate; they reinforce each other, making the pain experience more intense and persistent.

Recognizing these loops isn't just about identifying what's wrong—it's about seeing where you can intervene. By focusing on small, intentional actions, it is possible to disrupt these loops and create ripples of positive change that cascade across all systems.

Reflection Prompt: *Think about the last time your pain felt worse. What biological, psychological, or social factors might have been amplifying it? Could a small change in one area have made a difference?*

To make sense of how these amplifiers interact, imagine a simple diagram of three interconnected systems—biological, psychological, and social—each feeding into the others. When one system is disrupted, the others follow suit, creating a self-reinforcing cycle. For instance, physical pain can lead to sleepless nights, heightening emotional distress and driving social withdrawal. This isolation further elevates stress hormones and inflammation, locking the body and mind into a persistent state of pain. The cycle becomes self-sustaining, locking you in a state where pain perpetuates itself.

But just as these loops can amplify pain, they can also amplify healing. A small improvement in one area can ripple outward, affecting the others in unexpected ways. Learning to calm the nervous system, for example, might help you sleep better, which can improve your mood and give you the energy to reconnect with others. These small changes accumulate, creating new, positive feedback loops that support resilience and healing.

MASTERING CHRONIC PAIN

The Pain Amplification Feedback Loop

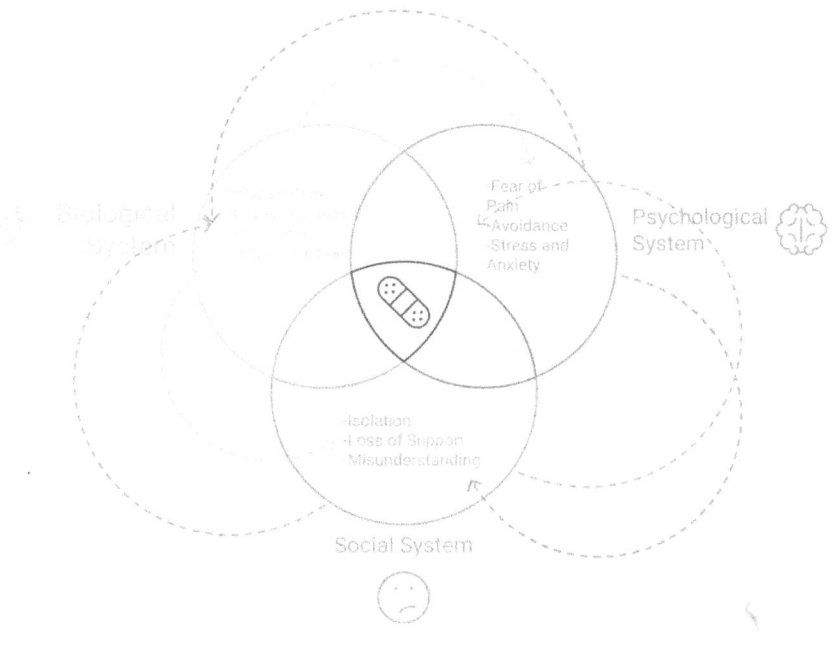

"What triggers seem to make your pain louder? Think about how your body reacts, what thoughts come up, or how your interactions with others feel. Write down one area where you notice the biggest ripple effect."

193

SIDEBAR

Take Action: Breaking the Amplification Loop

To break the amplification loop, try one of the following:

1. Biological: Try a guided progressive relaxation exercise. Start with your toes and work your way up, tensing and relaxing each muscle group. Notice how this calms your body.
2. Psychological: Write a letter to yourself as if you were a supportive friend, acknowledging your pain and encouraging yourself with words of kindness.
3. Social: Schedule a short walk with a friend or family member. Moving together creates connection and adds physical benefits.

Each action creates a ripple effect, gradually shifting the cycle from pain to resilience.

BREAKING THE CYCLE: TRANSFORMING AMPLIFIERS INTO RESILIENCE BUILDERS

Once you understand how amplifiers sustain chronic pain, the next step is learning to disrupt them. Amplifiers aren't inherently negative—they're simply systems that reflect the inputs they receive. When pain and stress dominate, amplifiers create destructive feedback loops. But when resilience-building practices are introduced, these same systems can be harnessed to amplify healing.

Think of amplifiers as ripples in a pond. Dropping a single stone into the water creates a ripple that spreads outward, touching everything in its path. In the same way, a small, intentional change—like improving sleep or practicing mindfulness—can set off a chain reaction that affects your entire system. For example, better sleep can calm the nervous system, reduce inflammation, and improve emotional resilience. This, in turn, can strengthen your relationships and reduce feelings of isolation, amplifying the positive effects across all areas of life.

The beauty of this process lies in its simplicity. You don't need to overhaul everything at once. Instead, focus on one manageable change, allowing it to ripple outward and create momentum.

Affirmation: *Every small change I make is a step toward breaking the pain cycle. I have the power to create ripples of resilience.*

To transform amplifiers into resilience builders, the Peak Resilience Method emphasizes addressing the biological, psychological, and social systems simultaneously. This holistic approach ensures that each system supports the others, creating a feedback loop that amplifies healing and strengthens resilience. By working within this framework, even small changes can ripple outward across all areas of your life.

For instance:

- A calming practice like diaphragmatic breathing can quiet the nervous system, reducing both physical pain and emotional stress.
- Reframing negative thoughts about pain can boost motivation, making it easier to engage in social activities that lift your spirits.
- Strengthening connections with loved ones can reduce feelings of isolation, calming the body's stress response and enhancing your capacity to heal.

Think about one small change you've made in the past—whether it was adding a healthy habit or reaching out to someone for support. What ripple effects did it have on other areas of your life? Reflect on how even small steps can create meaningful change and consider how this principle might apply to breaking the pain cycle.

SIDEBAR

Take Action: Transforming Your Amplifiers

To begin shifting your feedback loops toward resilience, try these simple practices:

1. Biological Amplifier: Start with a 5-minute diaphragmatic breathing exercise. Sit comfortably, place one hand on your belly, and take slow, deep breaths, feeling your belly rise as you inhale and fall as you exhale. This activates the Vagus nerve, calming the nervous system and reducing pain sensitivity.

2. Psychological Amplifier: Practice reframing a common negative thought about your pain. For instance, if you often think, "This pain controls my life," replace it with, "I am taking steps to manage this pain and regain control."

3. Social Amplifier: Reach out to one trusted friend or family member. Share how you're feeling, even briefly, to begin reducing feelings of isolation. This simple act of connection

can help soothe emotional distress and strengthen your support network.

Each step may seem small, but each one plants the seed for larger changes. By consistently introducing resilience-building practices into your daily life, you begin to rewrite the story of your pain—replacing the loops of stress and dysfunction with loops of healing and growth.

RESILIENCE AS A POSITIVE AMPLIFIER

The Peak Resilience Method shows how the same systems that sustain chronic pain can also be harnessed to amplify healing and resilience. By addressing your body, mind, and relationships holistically, these practices work together to shift you into states that support recovery and renewal. This is not just about managing symptoms; it's about creating a foundation where healing becomes possible, as we'll see in the next several chapters.

To turn amplifiers into resilience builders, target all three areas—biological, psychological, and social—one step at a time. Think of these steps as tools you can adapt to fit your life, building a personalized approach to healing.

Biological Resilience (chapter thirteen): Start with practices that calm your nervous system and reduce inflammation. For example, prioritizing hydration throughout the day supports cellular function and eases inflammation, while engaging in gentle, rhythmic movement—such as walking or light stretching—releases tension and boosts circulation.

Psychological Resilience (chapter fourteen): Work on rewiring your thoughts to disrupt negative patterns. Begin with something as simple as a daily mantra: "I am learning to manage my pain and build my resilience." This repetition isn't just motivational—it starts to create new neural connections that weaken fear and reinforce hope.

Social Resilience (chapter fifteen): Strengthen your connections by creating rituals of interaction. Even something as simple as sitting down for dinner with your family or scheduling a weekly call with a friend can break the cycle of isolation. These small rituals become anchors of support.

SUSTAINING MOMENTUM: CONSISTENCY CREATES TRANSFORMATION

The path to resilience is not about perfection or dramatic shifts—it's about taking small, deliberate actions that add up over time. Positive feedback loops grow stronger through repetition, gradually replacing cycles of pain with cycles of healing. Each small action builds on the last, helping your body, mind, and relationships work together more effectively.

The power of resilience lies in making it a habit. The actions you take today—no matter how small—lay the groundwork for long-term change. Consider how small, repeated steps ripple outward:

- Practicing progressive relaxation for ten minutes each evening trains your body to release tension, preparing you for deeper, restorative sleep.
- Joining a weekly community class—whether for yoga, book discussions, or creative projects—offers both physical and social benefits, reducing isolation and improving mood.
- Exploring anti-inflammatory snacks, like berries or nuts, integrates better nutrition into your daily routine without overhauling your diet all at once.

These practices don't have to feel overwhelming. The secret to transformation lies in their cumulative effect.

"What's one resilience habit that's felt good to you recently? How could you double its impact this week—by practicing more often or with greater focus?"

SIDEBAR

Take Action: The Next-Level Step

To strengthen your momentum, consider expanding on practices you've already started:

1. If you're calming your nervous system: Try a "five senses grounding exercise" to calm your nervous system. Name one thing you see, hear, feel, smell, and taste around you to focus on the present moment.
2. If you're working on nutrition: Prepare a batch of herbal tea (like chamomile or ginger) to sip throughout the day, reducing inflammation and stress.
3. If you're reconnecting socially: Join a virtual or in-person support group where others understand and share your pain journey.

Each step helps you weave resilience into your daily life, creating a routine that feels manageable yet impactful.

SIDEBAR

Take Action: Celebrate Your Progress

Sustaining resilience begins with celebrating small wins. Chronic pain often sharpens attention on difficulties, but each moment of progress—no matter how small—reminds you that healing is possible. Maybe your pain eased slightly after a breathing session, or perhaps a conversation with a friend left you feeling supported. These moments matter.

Consider creating a Progress Tracker to celebrate your wins. This can be as simple as jotting down three things you accomplished each day, no matter how small. For instance:

- "Did my breathing exercise before bed."
- "Added turmeric to my lunch."
- "Responded to a friend's text."

Over time, these records provide motivation and proof that change is happening, even when it feels gradual.

AMPLIFYING RESILIENCE, ONE STEP AT A TIME

Resilience grows through small, intentional actions that ripple outward, transforming your experience of pain. Though chronic pain can feel overwhelming, every positive choice you make creates momentum toward healing and hope. By understanding how amplifiers work and using them to your advantage, you can disrupt the loops that sustain pain and create new patterns of healing.

Every moment you choose to act—whether it's practicing mindfulness, reaching out for connection, or making a healthier choice for your body—you're amplifying your resilience. These actions may seem small, but they build on each other, strengthening the systems that support your recovery. Over time, they become the foundation of a life where pain no longer defines you.

Think of this chapter as your entrance into your toolkit for change. The steps you take don't have to be perfect or even consistent at first; they simply need to begin. In the next chapter, we'll take a moment to revisit strategies specific to addressing trauma, which can be a huge culprit from preventing us from amplifying resilience and keeping us stuck in patterns of pain. And then we'll move specifically into tactics for amplifying biological, psychological, and social resilience to chronic pain.

With each step forward, you're proving to yourself that resilience isn't just possible—it's happening. The pain might still be there, but its power to control your life is diminishing with every positive choice you make.

CHAPTER 12
ANOTHER LOOK AT COPING WITH TRAUMA

The relationship between trauma and chronic pain is not one-sided. As we established through Andre's story in chapter eight, trauma amplifies pain, but pain can also reinforce trauma, creating a vicious cycle that feels impossible to escape. Understanding this feedback loop is crucial for breaking free and building resilience. With that in mind, in this chapter, we'll specifically look at tools you can add to your resilience toolkit that address or relate to trauma and the pain-stress feedback loop it's notorious for reinforcing.

TRAUMA AMPLIFIES PAIN

Unresolved trauma changes how the nervous system perceives and processes pain. When the brain becomes conditioned to expect danger, it remains on high alert, which amplifies pain signals. For example, trauma can lead to neuroinflammation, a state where the brain and spinal cord are flooded with inflammatory chemicals that heighten the intensity of pain sensations. Additionally, the experience of pain itself can trigger fear, which only strengthens the brain's alarm response. If a previous traumatic event involved significant pain—such as an injury, surgery, or illness—new episodes of pain can reawaken the brain's memory of that trauma, making current pain feel far worse.

PAIN TRIGGERS TRAUMA MEMORIES

This connection is not just physical. Pain carries an emotional weight that can resurface old wounds. Chronic pain often acts as a trigger for trauma memories, especially if those experiences were tied to feelings of helplessness or fear. When pain reminds the brain of past distress, it can lead to heightened stress responses, such as muscle tension or the release of stress hormones like cortisol. This emotional flooding reinforces the feedback loop, making it harder to separate the sensations of pain from the emotions tied to trauma.

THE SOCIAL DIMENSION OF THE FEEDBACK LOOP

Isolation often worsens this cycle. Trauma and pain can both lead to withdrawing from others, whether because of shame, fear of being misunderstood, or lack of energy to connect. But isolation increases stress and heightens pain sensitivity. Without social connection, the body struggles to regulate stress hormones and calm the nervous system. Relationships that provide safety and trust are essential for buffering the effects of trauma and pain. Without them, the cycle of pain and trauma can spiral further.

BREAKING THE FEEDBACK LOOP

Breaking this feedback loop may feel daunting, but it's possible. A critical first step is focusing on safety—creating environments, routines, or relationships where you feel physically and emotionally secure. This might mean spending time with a trusted friend, developing soothing rituals at home, or working with a trauma-informed therapist who can help you navigate the connection between pain and trauma. Every small step toward safety helps calm the brain's alarm system, reducing the intensity of both pain and trauma over time.

To understand the relationship between your pain and trauma, it can be helpful to reflect on the patterns they create. Do your pain episodes bring up emotions or memories? Are there moments when your pain feels tied to past experiences or feelings? Mapping these connections can help you visualize the feedback loop and identify areas where you might disrupt it. For instance, you might notice that moments of fear or isolation intensify your pain, while reaching out to someone or practicing calming techniques helps ease the cycle. Even small changes, like pausing to take deep breaths during a pain episode or sharing your feelings with a supportive person, can begin to weaken the loop.

The pain-trauma feedback loop isn't permanent. Each time you reduce stress or soothe your nervous system, you take a step toward breaking the cycle. With patience and persistence, these efforts can help untangle the connection between pain and trauma, opening the door to healing.

How does your pain connect to emotions or memories? Are there moments when your pain feels tied to past experiences or feelings?

SIDEBAR

Take Action: Mapping the Feedback Loop

This exercise helps you identify patterns where pain and trauma reinforce each other.

Step 1: On a piece of paper, draw a circle and write "Pain" in the center. Around it, write down any emotions, memories, or behaviors that seem connected to your pain (e.g., fear, isolation, or past injuries).

Step 2: Draw lines between these items to show how they interact. For example:

- Pain → Fear → Stress → More Pain.

Step 3: Look for one small change you could make to disrupt this cycle, such as practicing deep breathing during moments of pain or reaching out to someone for support.

This visualization can help you see the connections between pain and trauma and begin to untangle them.

HEALING TRAUMA TO BREAK THE CYCLE OF PAIN

Breaking free from the trauma-pain feedback loop requires more than willpower—it demands a compassionate and intentional approach to healing. Trauma affects the very foundation of your body's internal systems, but these patterns can be rewired. Healing begins with safety and trust, essential elements for calming your nervous system and opening the door to recovery.

THE ROLE OF SAFETY AND TRUST

Trauma leaves your body in a state of constant vigilance, scanning for threats even when you are not in danger. To begin healing, you need to signal to your brain and body that it is safe to relax. This process starts by creating both physical and emotional safety.

Physical safety might involve setting boundaries to protect your energy or cultivating environments that feel calm and soothing, such as your home or a favorite outdoor space. Emotional safety often requires trust, whether in relationships or with yourself. Trust-building can be as simple as following through on commitments to yourself, like pausing for self-care when needed or practicing kindness in your inner dialogue.

Trust also extends to relationships. Trauma often makes it difficult to rely on others, but supportive and understanding connections are a powerful tool for healing. A trusted friend, family member, or therapist can help you feel seen and understood, reducing the isolation and fear that feed the trauma-pain cycle.

THE BIOPSYCHOSOCIAL MODEL AND TRAUMA WORK

Healing trauma is not just about emotional release—it involves working across all dimensions of your well-being: biological, psychological, and social. This integrated approach ensures that every layer of the trauma-pain cycle is addressed.

Biological Healing: Practices like mindfulness, restorative movement, and Vagus nerve stimulation help calm your nervous system and reduce neuroinflammation.

Psychological Healing: Cognitive reframing, journaling, and trauma-informed therapy can help you process painful memories and rewire negative thought patterns.

Social Healing: Building or rebuilding trust in safe relationships fosters connection and helps regulate stress responses.

Each pillar reinforces the others. For example, calming your nervous system makes it easier to think clearly and connect with others, while supportive relationships help lower stress and inflammation. This interconnection is central to the Peak Resilience Method.

What feels safe to you? Is there a person, place, or practice that helps you feel grounded and secure? How might trust—whether with yourself or others—play a role in your healing process?

SIDEBAR

Take Action: Creating a Safety Toolkit

This exercise helps you identify tools and practices that signal safety to your body and mind.

1. Identify Your Safety Cues: Think about what makes you feel calm and safe. It could be a quiet room, a favorite blanket, or a loved one's voice. Write down three to five things that help you feel secure.
2. Build Your Toolkit: Gather physical items or reminders of these safety cues. For example:
   - Keep a photo of a comforting place or person nearby.
   - Use an essential oil or fabric with a soothing scent.
   - Create a playlist of calming music.
3. Use Your Toolkit: When you feel overwhelmed, reach for one or more items in your toolkit to help regulate your nervous system and ground yourself.

PRACTICAL STRATEGIES FOR HEALING TRAUMA AND BUILDING RESILIENCE

Healing trauma and building resilience require a combination of professional support and self-guided practices. Each strategy offers tools to process emotions, calm the body's stress response, and foster long-term recovery. Together, these approaches provide a foundation for breaking the trauma-pain cycle.

Professional Help: Evidence-Based Therapies

Trauma-informed therapies offer structured methods for addressing the emotional and physical effects of trauma. By processing painful memories, calming the nervous system, and reframing negative thought patterns, these therapies help restore balance and resilience.

Eye Movement Desensitization and Reprocessing (EMDR): This therapy uses guided eye movements to help reprocess traumatic memories, reducing their emotional intensity and relieving stress.

Somatic Experiencing: A body-centered approach that helps release trauma stored in physical tension and restores a sense of safety and ease.

Cognitive Behavioral Therapy (CBT): This method helps identify and reframe negative thoughts linked to trauma, offering practical tools to reduce fear and improve emotional regulation.

Internal Family Systems (IFS): IFS therapy explores the "parts" of yourself that may have developed in response to trauma, such as protective or reactive parts. By connecting with these parts compassionately, you can create greater inner harmony and self-compassion.

These therapies work best when guided by licensed professionals with expertise in trauma care.

Emerging Research: Psychedelic-Assisted Therapies

Though not yet widely available or approved for clinical use in the U.S., psychedelic-assisted therapies are an exciting area of research for trauma and PTSD. Early studies at institutions like Johns Hopkins and Imperial College London suggest that substances such as MDMA and psilocybin may help individuals process trauma and promote emotional healing. These therapies remain experimental but highlight the growing understanding of trauma's complexity and the innovative approaches being explored for recovery.

Self-Guided Practices: Tools for Everyday Healing

While professional therapies provide structured guidance, self-guided practices empower you to take an active role in your healing journey. These techniques are accessible and can be integrated into daily life:

Mindfulness: Practicing mindfulness, even for a few minutes a day, can help you stay present and disengage from trauma-driven worry or fear. Over time, mindfulness reduces stress hormones and strengthens emotional regulation.

Journaling: Writing about your thoughts and feelings offers a private, safe space to process emotions and recognize patterns in your responses to trauma and pain. Reflecting on your progress can also provide encouragement.

Grounding Exercises: Techniques like the 5-4-3-2-1 method anchor you in the present moment. Identifying five things you see, four you can touch, three you hear, two you smell, and one you taste can help calm overwhelming emotions.

Restorative Movement: Gentle practices like yoga, tai chi, or simple stretching release tension stored in the body and help reset your nervous system, promoting balance and resilience.

Reconnecting with Others: Trauma often leads to isolation, but social connection is one of the most powerful tools for healing. Trusted relationships provide emotional support and help regulate stress responses, while shared experiences in groups or communities can rebuild trust.

When reconnecting, it's important to choose relationships and environments that feel safe and supportive. Avoid spaces that promote negativity or invalidate your experiences, as these can reinforce feelings of disconnection. If direct interaction feels overwhelming, online communities or trauma-informed support groups can provide an accessible starting point.

Which of these strategies feels most approachable to you? How might you begin incorporating one or two into your routine this week?

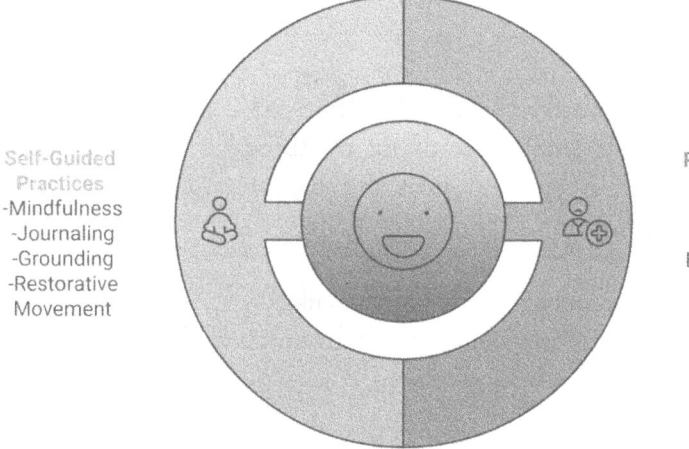

Healing Trauma Approaches

Self-Guided Practices
-Mindfulness
-Journaling
-Grounding
-Restorative Movement

Professional Therapies
-EMDR
-Somatic Experiencing
-CBT
-IFS

SIDEBAR

Take Acton: Building Your Personal Healing Plan

This exercise helps you combine professional and self-guided strategies into a personalized plan for resilience.

- Identify a Professional Option: Research local trauma-informed therapists or clinics offering therapies like EMDR, CBT, or IFS. Set a goal to reach out to one.
- Choose Two Self-Guided Practices: Select two techniques, such as mindfulness or journaling, to try over the next week. Schedule a specific time to practice each.
- Track Your Progress: Use a journal or app to reflect on how these strategies affect your emotions, stress levels, and pain. Note what feels helpful and where adjustments might be needed.

TURNING PAIN INTO PURPOSE

No one should have to experience trauma. It leaves a profound and lasting mark, shaping how we see ourselves and the world around us. While the pain of trauma is undeniable, healing offers a path to transformation. It creates space for growth, connection, and a renewed sense of purpose, enabling you to move beyond survival and rediscover what truly matters in your life.

For many, trauma can feel like a permanent barrier, a wound that defines their identity. But healing transforms trauma from an obstacle into an opportunity for growth. This shift doesn't erase the pain—it reframes it, revealing the strength and resilience that have carried you through.

Research shows that people who recover from trauma often experience post-traumatic growth, a process where they gain new perspectives, resilience, and a deeper appreciation for life. This growth doesn't diminish the difficulty of trauma; instead, it highlights the potential for healing to lead to personal transformation.

Healing also helps you reconnect with what matters most. Trauma often traps you in survival mode, narrowing your focus to immediate challenges. But as you recover, you begin to notice a renewed interest in activities you once loved, greater clarity about your values, and a deeper sense of connection to others. Trauma may have disconnected you from these aspects of yourself, but recovery creates the space needed to reengage with what brings you joy. This process begins with small, intentional steps. You might start by journaling about your values, reaching out to a supportive friend, or exploring an activity that feels meaningful. Over time, these small steps can help you move beyond pain and rediscover your purpose.

Turning Pain into Purpose

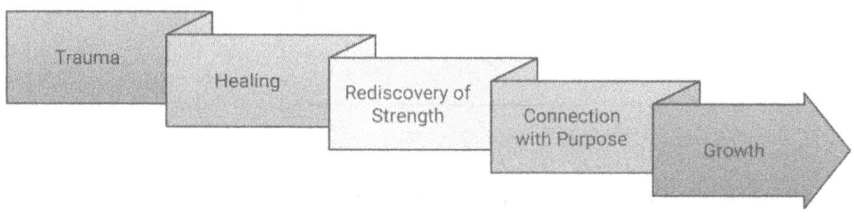

If your pain no longer held you back, what would you want to do? How could your experiences shape the way you connect with others or pursue your goals?

SIDEBAR

Take Action: Rediscovering Your Purpose

This exercise helps you reconnect with what matters most:

1. Reflect on Joy: Write down activities, relationships, or moments that have brought you joy in the past. Don't filter your thoughts—just let them flow.
2. Identify Your Values: Ask yourself: What truly matters to me? What kind of person do I want to be? Write down three to five core values that feel most meaningful.

Take a Small Step: Choose one thing from your list of joys or values and commit to taking a tangible step toward it this week. For example, if connecting with nature brings you peace, take a short walk outside or plan a visit to a park.

MOVING BEYOND TRAUMA

Trauma may shape your story, but much like Andre came to learn in chapter eight, it does not define you. Healing is not about forgetting or erasing the past—it's about reclaiming your power and finding a way to thrive in spite of what you've been through. Through the steps outlined in this chapter—addressing the roots of trauma, calming your body's responses, and reconnecting with yourself and others—you are already building resilience. Each small action you take is a declaration that your life can be bigger than the pain, richer than the past, and filled with the purpose you deserve to rediscover.

Imagine a version of yourself no longer burdened by the weight of trauma or pain. What passions might you pursue? What relationships would you nurture? What kind of impact could you have on the world? The answers to these questions aren't just dreams—they're the vision of a life transformed, made possible by the choices you make today.

Healing from trauma is a journey, not a destination. The tools you've explored in this chapter aren't one-time activities. Revisiting the ACEs questionnaire, the body scan, or your personal healing plan as you progress can deepen your understanding and support your growth. Each time you return to these practices, you'll uncover new insights and build on your resilience.

Some days will be easier than others, but every step forward matters. Your story is still unfolding, and with every act of courage and self-compassion, you're shaping a future filled with growth, connection, and meaning.

CHAPTER 13
REBUILDING AND AMPLIFYING BIOLOGICAL RESILIENCE

As we've covered, for many living with chronic pain—like Lisa, who we met earlier, and perhaps you—traditional medical treatments like medications, injections, or physical therapy provide important relief. These tools often play a key role in managing pain and improving function. But if you've ever felt like these treatments aren't enough on their own, or like their effects don't last, you're not alone.

That's where resilience comes in. Biological resilience, in particular, strengthens your body's foundation, making it more adaptable to the challenges of chronic pain. By calming the nervous system, reducing inflammation, and improving your body's energy production, you create the conditions for deeper healing. This doesn't replace the medical tools you're already using—it enhances their effectiveness, helping them work better for you.

In earlier chapters, we discussed how chronic pain creates internal system sabotage—a state where the nervous, immune, and endocrine systems become stuck in patterns that sustain pain. In this chapter, we'll focus on practical ways to start reversing that process through biological resilience. Now, as you start building the biological toolkit for your Resilience Code, we'll focus on practical ways to start reversing that process through biological resilience in five key areas:

Calming the Nervous System: Shifting from "fight or flight" to "rest and repair."

Reducing Inflammation: Simple, sustainable changes to lower chronic inflammation.

Supporting Cellular Health: Boosting energy production through gentle movement and targeted nutrition.

Restoring Gut Health: Strengthening the gut-brain connection for better balance.

Improving Sleep: Practical steps to enhance restorative sleep.

Each section will include actionable steps you can start implementing today, along with prompts to help you personalize the practices to fit your life. These strategies are designed to be simple yet impactful, creating a foundation for recovery without feeling overwhelming.

Affirmation: *Every small choice I make to support my body builds my resilience. Progress is a journey, and each step counts.*

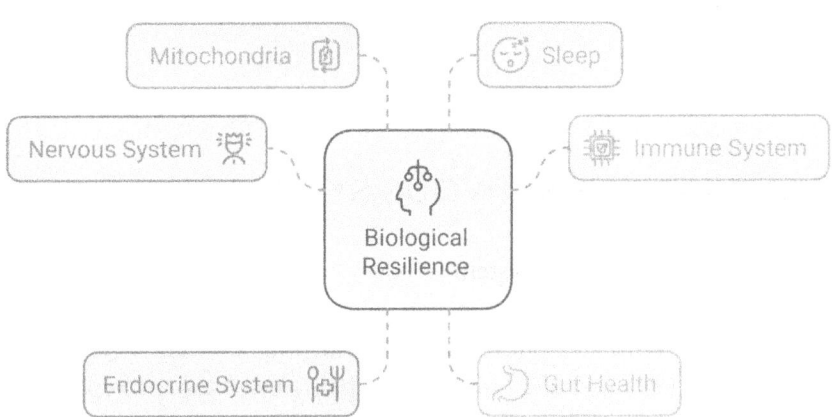

> **Key Takeaways for Biological Resilience:**
>
> - Small Steps Matter: Start with manageable habits, like adding one anti-inflammatory food or practicing deep breathing for five minutes daily.
> - Build Momentum: Tracking your wins, no matter how small, reinforces progress.
> - Integrated Approach: Combining biological, psychological, and social resilience amplifies healing.

SIDEBAR

Take Action: Start with Small Changes

- Nervous System: Try 4-7-8 breathing to calm your mind and body. Inhale for 4 seconds, hold for 7, and exhale for 8. Repeat 3–5 times.
- Inflammation: Swap sugary snacks for nuts or a piece of fruit.
- Sleep: Turn off screens 30 minutes before bedtime and read a book instead or listen to a sleep meditation.

CALMING THE NERVOUS SYSTEM

Your autonomic nervous system (ANS) works behind the scenes to regulate key functions like breathing, heart rate, and digestion. It's designed to run on autopilot, seamlessly shifting between "fight or flight" mode (when you're stressed or in pain) and "rest and repair" mode (when your body heals and restores itself).

Chronic pain, however, often traps the ANS in "fight or flight," keeping your body in a constant state of nervous system activation. This can amplify pain signals, increase tension, and drain your energy reserves.

The good news? With simple, intentional techniques, you can nudge your nervous system back into balance. By being mindful of your state —whether you feel calm, tense, or somewhere in between—you can begin to use these practices to promote relaxation and support your body's healing processes.

KEY ACTIONS TO CALM THE NERVOUS SYSTEM

1. Practice Progressive Muscle Relaxation (PMR)

Why It Works

PMR interrupts the cycle of tension and stress reinforced by chronic pain. By tensing and releasing muscle groups, you send signals to your brain that it's safe to let go of tension. Research shows that PMR reduces cortisol (the body's primary stress hormone) and can decrease pain sensitivity by calming overactive pain pathways.

What to Do

1. Find a quiet space to sit or lie down comfortably.
2. Start with your feet: Tense the muscles in your toes and hold for 5 seconds, then release.
3. Move upward—calves, thighs, abdomen, arms, and face—tensing each group for 5 seconds and then releasing.
4. Breathe deeply as you relax each area, focusing on the sensation of release.

Try This

Practice PMR before bedtime to improve sleep quality and reduce pain flare-ups at night.

"Where in your body do you feel the most tension right now? Could you focus on releasing those areas with PMR today?"

---

2. Shift Your Breathing

When Lisa first learned about diaphragmatic breathing form us, she thought it sounded too simple to help with his chronic pain. But one afternoon, after a stressful day at work, she gave it a try. Sitting in her car, she placed one hand on her chest and the other on her belly, following the rise and fall of her breath. After just a few minutes, Lisa noticed her shoulders had relaxed, her racing thoughts had slowed, and her pain felt a little less intense. It became a daily ritual that gave her a sense of control in overwhelming moments.

Why It Works

Deep breathing activates the Vagus nerve, a key player in your parasympathetic nervous system, which helps shift your body from "fight or flight" to "rest and repair." Research shows that prolonged exhales reduce heart rate, lower blood pressure, and decrease overall stress, making breathing exercises an accessible and powerful tool for pain management.

What to Do

1. Sit or lie down comfortably. Place one hand on your stomach and one on your chest.
2. Inhale deeply through your nose for 4 counts, letting your stomach rise.
3. Hold your breath for 7 counts, noticing the stillness.
4. Exhale slowly and completely through your mouth for 8 counts, feeling your stomach fall.
5. Repeat this pattern for 5–10 breaths.

Pro Tip

If 4-7-8 feels difficult, start with a shorter ratio (e.g., 4-4-6) and gradually increase your exhale length as it becomes easier.

Enhancing Your Practice with Technology

External Vagus Nerve Stimulation

Technology can complement breathing exercises by electrically stimulating the Vagus nerve. Devices designed for auricular Vagus nerve stimulation (gentle electrical stimulation of the ear's Vagus nerve branches) or vagus nerve stimulation along the neck are non-invasive tools that help promote relaxation.

What to Know

- Devices are increasingly accessible for home use but should be discussed with your healthcare provider before trying.
- Pairing Vagus nerve stimulation with breathing exercises may enhance the calming effects on the nervous system.

> *"How often do you think about your breathing? Could tools like Vagus nerve stimulation or controlled breathing fit into your routine?"*

3. Embrace Restorative Movement

Why It Works

Gentle activities like yoga, tai chi, or even simple stretching combine movement with mindfulness, calming the nervous system while improving circulation and flexibility. These practices can also release endorphins—your body's natural painkillers—and regulate cortisol levels, helping to ease pain.

What to Do

- Start small with 5–10 minutes of movement each day. If yoga or tai chi feels intimidating, try basic stretches:
  - Reach your arms toward the ceiling for a full-body stretch.
  - Rotate your neck gently from side to side.
  - Roll your shoulders to release tension.
- Pair your movements with slow, steady breathing for added relaxation.

Pro Tip

Choose a time of day when movement feels most accessible—whether it's a morning stretch to wake up your body or an evening cooldown to unwind.

> *"What's one movement or stretch you already enjoy? Could you add it to your daily routine to support your nervous system?"*

Your nervous system may feel stuck on autopilot, but small, consistent practices can help you regain control. By regularly practicing these techniques—even for just a few minutes a day—you can create a calmer state that supports healing. Start with one strategy today—whether it's a few deep breaths, a muscle relaxation exercise, or a short stretch—and notice how your body begins to respond.

REDUCING INFLAMMATION AND IMMUNE OVERACTIVATION

Inflammation is a natural part of the body's healing process. When you sprain an ankle or catch a cold, your immune system creates inflammation to fight off harmful invaders and repair damage. But in chronic pain, this helpful process can get stuck in overdrive, leading to ongoing inflammation that damages tissues, amplifies pain signals, and hinders recovery.

For many, managing this inflammation has meant relying on nonsteroidal anti-inflammatory drugs (NSAIDs) like ibuprofen or naproxen. While NSAIDs can provide short-term relief, chronic use can lead to side effects such as gastrointestinal issues, kidney strain, or even cardiovascular risks. This is why it's helpful to explore complementary strategies that reduce inflammation naturally, either alongside NSAIDs or as alternatives where appropriate.

Emerging options like curcumin—a compound found in turmeric—and low-dose naltrexone (LDN) are gaining attention for their potential anti-inflammatory and pain-modulating effects. These tools aren't one-size-fits-all, but for some, they represent valuable options to discuss with a healthcare provider.

By making small, consistent changes to your lifestyle—especially in how you eat, drink, and manage stress—you can help calm this immune overactivation. This section focuses on practical, sustainable steps to reduce inflammation and create a healthier internal environment for healing.

KEY ACTIONS TO REDUCE INFLAMMATION

1. Add Anti-Inflammatory Foods to Your Plate

Why It Works

Certain foods naturally contain compounds that reduce inflammation, like omega-3 fatty acids, antioxidants, and phytonutrients. Regularly incorporating these foods into your diet helps counteract chronic inflammation and supports overall healing.

What to Do

- Add at least one anti-inflammatory ingredient to each meal. Examples include:
    - **Breakfast**: Top your oatmeal with fresh berries or sprinkle flaxseeds into your yogurt.
    - **Lunch**: Add a handful of spinach to your sandwich or enjoy a salad with olive oil dressing.
    - **Dinner**: Incorporate fatty fish (like salmon) or roasted vegetables like broccoli or sweet potatoes.

Pro Tip

When choosing fish, prioritize wild-caught salmon over farm-raised when possible. Wild-caught salmon typically contains fewer contaminants like antibiotics and has higher levels of omega-3 fatty acids. If you're consuming big deepwater fish like tuna or swordfish, be mindful of mercury levels—limit intake to once a week to avoid overexposure.

Curcumin (Turmeric)

Why It Works

Curcumin, the active compound in turmeric, has been shown in studies to reduce inflammation by inhibiting inflammatory markers like cytokines. It also has antioxidant properties, which help protect cells from damage caused by chronic inflammation.

How to Use It

- Include turmeric in your cooking—add it to soups, stews, or roasted vegetables for both flavor and potential benefits.
- Consider taking a curcumin supplement if advised by your healthcare provider. Not all curcumin supplements are absorbed equally, so the formulation likely matters. Look for options designed to improve bioavailability, such as those combined with black pepper extract (piperine) or advanced absorption technologies.

Pro Tip

Curcumin may not work for everyone, and its effects are often seen over weeks, not days. It's best used as part of a long-term strategy for inflammation management.

2. **Stay Hydrated**

Why It Works

Water is essential for flushing toxins, reducing inflammation, and supporting your body's natural repair processes. Dehydration, on the other hand, can exacerbate inflammation and amplify pain.

What to Do

- Start your morning with a full glass of water before coffee or tea.
- Carry a reusable water bottle throughout the day and sip regularly.
- Aim for 8–10 cups of water daily, adjusting based on your activity level and environment.

Enhance This with Technology

Consider using tools like:

- **Smart Water Bottles**: Devices like the HidrateSpark track your hydration in real time and sync with your phone.
- **Hydration Apps**: Apps such as Plant Nanny or WaterMinder send reminders to drink water and track your daily intake visually.

Pro Tip

If plain water feels boring, infuse it with fresh lemon, cucumber, or mint for a refreshing twist.

3. **Limit Pro-Inflammatory Triggers**

Why It Works

While adding anti-inflammatory foods is key, it's also helpful to limit items that fuel inflammation, such as processed sugars, trans fats, and refined carbohydrates. Small, gradual adjustments can significantly lower your body's inflammatory load.

What to Do

- Start by reducing one pro-inflammatory food in your diet. For instance:
    - Swap sugary drinks for herbal teas or water.
    - Replace fried snacks with raw nuts or seeds.
    - Choose whole-grain bread over white bread.

Try This

Make one swap at a time so the changes feel manageable and sustainable.

Low-Dose Naltrexone (LDN)

Why It Works

LDN, a lower-dose formulation of a drug traditionally used to treat addiction, is being studied for its ability to reduce inflammation and modulate the immune system. It's thought to work by briefly blocking opioid receptors, which then triggers a rebound effect, increasing the body's production of endorphins and reducing inflammation.

How to Use It

- LDN is only available by prescription. If you're interested, talk to your healthcare provider about whether it might be a good option for your situation.
- Research suggests it's especially promising for conditions involving chronic inflammation, like fibromyalgia or autoimmune disorders.

Pro Tip

While LDN is still considered experimental for pain management, many patients and physicians are finding it to be a helpful adjunct to other treatments.

4. Manage Stress to Calm the Immune System

Why It Works

Chronic stress keeps your immune system in overdrive, releasing pro-inflammatory chemicals like cortisol and cytokines. Managing stress helps regulate these responses, giving your body space to heal.

What to Do

- Dedicate 5–10 minutes daily to a stress-relieving activity, such as:
  - Deep breathing or meditation.
  - Spending time in nature.
  - Journaling about positive moments from your day.

Pro Tip

We'll explore stress management in greater detail in the next chapter. For now, start with simple practices like spending a few minutes focusing on your breath or stepping outside for fresh air.

Reducing inflammation isn't about drastic changes—it's about making small, sustainable choices that add up over time. Whether it's adding colorful foods to your plate, drinking more water, or carving out moments to relax, every step you take helps calm your body's immune response and creates the conditions for healing.

Start with one change today. Over time, you'll build a lifestyle that not only reduces inflammation but also supports resilience in every part of your life.

SUPPORTING MITOCHONDRIA AND CELLULAR HEALTH

At the cellular level, your body's ability to heal and maintain resilience depends on energy—produced by tiny structures in your cells called mitochondria. These "powerhouses" are responsible for generating the energy your body needs for everything from repairing tissues to managing pain.

In chronic pain, mitochondrial function can decline, leading to fatigue, reduced cellular repair, and slower healing. By supporting mitochondrial health, you can boost your energy levels and help your body recover more effectively.

This section focuses on practical, science-backed steps to nurture your mitochondria, improve cellular function, and rebuild your energy reserves.

KEY ACTIONS TO SUPPORT MITOCHONDRIAL HEALTH

1. Incorporate Gentle Movement

Why It Works

Exercise stimulates mitochondrial activity by increasing oxygen delivery to cells and encouraging the production of new mitochondria. While intense workouts can be counterproductive for those in pain, gentle movement like walking, stretching, or yoga can enhance energy production without adding stress to the body.

What to Do

- Aim for 10–15 minutes of low-impact movement daily. Examples include:
    - A slow walk around your neighborhood.
    - Basic stretches to loosen tight muscles.
    - A gentle yoga flow or tai chi session.

Pro Tip

Try Zone 2 Exercise: Zone 2 exercise—moderate-intensity activity at 60–70% of your maximum heart rate—is particularly effective for mitochondria. At this level, your body primarily uses fat for fuel, which challenges mitochondria to work efficiently and multiply.

How to Identify Zone 2

- You should be able to carry on a conversation, but your breathing will feel slightly elevated.
- Examples include brisk walking, steady cycling, or leisurely swimming.

"What's one type of gentle or Zone 2 movement that feels good for your body? Could you try it for 10–15 minutes this week?"

---

2. Focus on Mitochondria-Friendly Nutrients

Why It Works

Mitochondria rely on specific nutrients to function efficiently, including:

- **B Vitamins**: Support energy metabolism.
- **Magnesium**: Essential for over 300 enzymatic reactions, including those in mitochondria.
- **Coenzyme Q10 (CoQ10)**: Helps mitochondria produce ATP, the body's energy currency.

What to Do

- Include foods rich in these nutrients:
  - B Vitamins: Leafy greens, eggs, lean meats.
  - Magnesium: Nuts, seeds, whole grains.
  - CoQ10: Fatty fish, organ meats, or supplements (consult your doctor).

Pro Tip

Not all supplements are created equal. Consult with a healthcare provider before starting any new supplementation to ensure it's safe and appropriate for you.

> *"Does your current diet include foods that support energy production? What's one nutrient-rich food you could add to your meals this week?"*

3. Embrace Sun Exposure and Red-Light Therapy

Why It Works

Light plays a critical role in mitochondrial health and energy production. Morning sunlight helps regulate your body's circadian rhythm, which synchronizes energy production and repair processes. Red light therapy, meanwhile, has shown promise in stimulating mitochondrial activity by enhancing ATP production—the energy currency of your cells.

What to Do

- **Morning Sunlight**: Spend 10–15 minutes outside in the

morning light to help align your circadian rhythm. No sunglasses needed but avoid staring directly at the sun.
- **Red Light Therapy**: If interested, talk to a healthcare provider about trying red light therapy. It's increasingly available for home use, but the evidence is still emerging, so use it as a complementary tool.

Pro Tip

Pair your morning sun exposure with a walk for double the benefits of light and movement.

"How often do you get direct sunlight during the day? Could you make a small effort to spend a few minutes outside each morning?"

4. Try Controlled Cold Exposure

Why It Works

Cold exposure activates brown fat, a type of fat tissue rich in mitochondria, which boosts energy production and reduces inflammation. It also stimulates norepinephrine release, improving focus and overall resilience.

What to Do

- **Cold Showers**: End your warm shower with 30 seconds of cold water, gradually increasing the duration as you adapt.
- **Cold Packs**: Apply a cold pack to your upper back or neck for a few minutes to experience mild effects.
- **Cold Plunge**: If you have access to an ice bath, aim for 1–2

minutes, but consult a professional if you're new to cold exposure.

Pro Tip

Always ease into cold exposure, especially if you have cardiovascular concerns. Discuss with your doctor if you're unsure whether it's right for you.

"What's one way you could safely try cold exposure this week? How might it benefit your energy or resilience?"

---

5. Get Consistent, Restorative Sleep

Why It Works

Your mitochondria do much of their repair work while you sleep. Poor sleep disrupts this process, leaving your cells less equipped to produce energy and manage inflammation.

What to Do

- Stick to a consistent sleep schedule, going to bed and waking up at the same time each day.
- Create a calming pre-sleep routine, such as reading, meditating, or listening to soft music.

Coming Up

We'll dive deeper into practical sleep strategies later in this chapter. For now, focus on creating consistency in your sleep schedule.

> *"What's one small change you could make tonight to improve your sleep quality?"*

Your mitochondria are small but mighty. By nurturing these cellular powerhouses with movement, light, nutrients, and rest, you can rebuild your energy and resilience. Start with just one of these practices today—whether it's stepping outside for morning sunlight, adding a nutrient-rich food to your plate, or trying a brief cold shower—and notice how your body responds.

Over time, these small shifts will help you feel more energized and ready to take on the next steps in your healing journey.

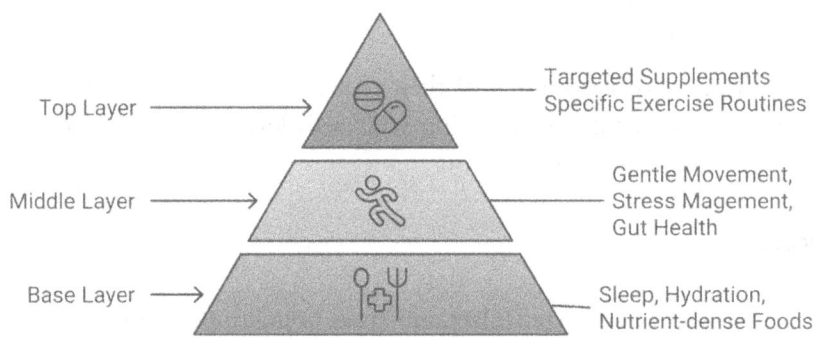

Biological Resilience: Building a Strong Foundation

- Top Layer → Targeted Supplements, Specific Exercise Routines
- Middle Layer → Gentle Movement, Stress Magement, Gut Health
- Base Layer → Sleep, Hydration, Nutrient-dense Foods

BALANCING THE ENDOCRINE SYSTEM: THE BODY'S MASTER REGULATOR

The endocrine system is like a master conductor in the symphony of your body's recovery. Through a network of hormones, it communicates with the nervous and immune systems, regulates cellular repair, and governs processes like sleep, metabolism, and energy production.

In chronic pain, this delicate balance is often disrupted. Stress, poor sleep, inflammation, and fatigue create a feedback loop that can suppress hormone production or throw key systems into overdrive. Cortisol, insulin, thyroid hormones, growth hormone, melatonin, and even sex hormones like testosterone and estrogen all play critical roles in either perpetuating pain or supporting resilience.

This interconnectedness is both a challenge and an opportunity. By making targeted changes to reduce stress, improve nutrition, and enhance sleep, you can begin to recalibrate your endocrine system. Small adjustments can ripple outward, creating balance across the web of your body's systems.

Key Hormones and What to Do

1. Cortisol: Manage Stress

The Problem

Chronic pain and stress elevate cortisol levels, which suppresses immune function, worsens inflammation, and disrupts energy and sleep.

What to Do

- Practice mindfulness, deep breathing, or progressive relaxation daily to calm the stress response.
- Incorporate short breaks into your day to reduce mental and physical tension.

"What's one small way you can reduce stress today? Could you pause for five deep breaths or take a short walk?"

2. Insulin: Balance Blood Sugar

The Problem

Insulin resistance, often triggered by inactivity and stress, leads to energy crashes and systemic inflammation.

What to Do

- Focus on balanced meals with protein, fiber, and healthy fats to stabilize blood sugar.
- Limit refined sugars and processed carbs, which spike insulin levels.

Try This

Swap a sugary snack for a handful of nuts or a piece of fruit with nut butter.

"What's one way you could make your next meal more balanced? Could you add a source of protein or fiber?"

---

3. Thyroid Hormones: Eat for Thyroid Health

The Problem

Dysregulated thyroid hormones result in fatigue, impaired metabolism, and reduced cellular repair.

What to Do

- Include selenium (e.g., Brazil nuts, seafood), iodine (e.g., seaweed, dairy), and zinc (e.g., seeds, shellfish) in your diet to support thyroid function.
- Emphasize healthy fats (e.g., avocados, olive oil, nuts) to support overall hormone production.

Pro Tip

A single Brazil nut provides your daily selenium needs—an easy addition to your routine!

"Is there a nutrient-rich food you enjoy that you could add to your meals this week?"

---

4. Melatonin and Growth Hormone: Optimize Sleep

The Problem

Disrupted sleep lowers melatonin and GH levels, reducing the body's ability to repair itself overnight.

What to Do

- Stick to a regular sleep schedule, and wind down with calming activities before bed.
- Reduce blue light exposure by turning off screens an hour before bedtime.

5. Testosterone and GH: Use Strength Training

The Problem

Chronic pain and inactivity lower testosterone and GH levels, slowing recovery and reducing muscle repair.

What to Do

- Strength training stimulates the release of testosterone and GH, which are crucial for building muscle, improving bone density, and supporting resilience. Start slow, especially if pain makes movement difficult. Begin with simple, low-resistance exercises like bodyweight squats or light dumbbells.
- Aim for 2-3 sessions per week. Start with light weights or bodyweight exercises to build confidence and prevent injury.
- A Note for Women: Testosterone isn't just a "male hormone." Women also produce testosterone, and it plays a vital role in muscle strength, bone health, and overall resilience. Incorporating strength training into your routine benefits everyone, regardless of gender.

Pro Tip

Pair strength training with Zone 2 cardio for balanced energy and recovery.

"What's one strength-building movement you feel confident trying this week?"

---

6. **Measure and Monitor Your Hormones**

The Problem

Hormonal imbalances can manifest in subtle ways, such as fatigue, mood changes, or poor recovery, and may require medical intervention.

What to Do

- Talk to your healthcare provider about measuring cortisol, insulin, thyroid hormones, testosterone, and other key levels.
- If needed, consider interventions like hormone replacement therapy (HRT) or targeted supplementation.

Pro Tip

Regular testing can help track progress and guide adjustments to your recovery plan.

Your endocrine system is a powerful web of interconnected messengers that regulate healing, energy, and resilience. Chronic pain may have disrupted this balance, but small, thoughtful changes—like managing stress, eating for hormonal health, improving sleep, and staying active—can help recalibrate your body's systems.

Every small step you take to restore hormonal balance supports your recovery journey, creating a ripple effect of healing across your entire body.

RESTORING GUT HEALTH FOR SYSTEMIC RESILIENCE

Your gut does far more than just digest food—as Lisa learned, it's a central hub for your overall health and resilience. Known as the gut-brain axis, the communication between your gut and your brain plays a critical role in regulating pain, mood, and immune function.

In chronic pain, disruptions in gut health—such as an imbalanced microbiome, leaky gut, or food sensitivities—can amplify pain signals, increase inflammation, and affect how your brain processes stress. Restoring gut health isn't just about improving digestion—it's about creating a foundation for resilience that supports every system in your body.

The 5 Rs of Gut Healing

A proven roadmap for improving gut health, the 5 Rs framework offers a structured approach to healing your digestive system:

1. Remove: Eliminate irritants like processed foods, alcohol, or specific food triggers identified through an elimination diet.
2. Replace: Add back digestive aids if needed, such as enzymes or bile salts, to support nutrient absorption.
3. Reinoculate: Rebuild your microbiome with probiotics and prebiotic-rich foods.
4. Repair: Strengthen the gut lining with nutrients like L-glutamine, zinc, or collagen.
5. Rebalance: Focus on lifestyle habits that promote gut health, such as managing stress and improving sleep.

This framework is flexible and can be adapted based on individual needs. Throughout this section, you'll find actionable steps tied to these principles.

Key Actions to Restore Gut Health

1. Add Probiotic and Prebiotic Foods

Why It Works

Probiotic foods introduce beneficial bacteria into your gut, while prebiotic foods feed these bacteria, helping them thrive. A balanced gut microbiome reduces inflammation, improves digestion, and influences your mood through the gut-brain axis.

What to Do

- Include probiotic-rich foods in your diet, such as:
    - Yogurt with live cultures.
    - Fermented foods like sauerkraut, kimchi, or miso.
    - Kefir or kombucha.
- Add prebiotic foods, which are high in fiber, like:
    - Garlic, onions, and leeks.
    - Bananas, apples, and asparagus.
    - Whole grains and legumes.

Pro Tip

If you're new to probiotics, start with small amounts to see how your body reacts. Some people may experience mild bloating as their gut adjusts.

"What's one probiotic or prebiotic food you already enjoy? Could you include it in a meal this week?"

2. Minimize Gut Irritants

Why It Works

Certain foods and medications can irritate the gut lining or disrupt the microbiome, worsening inflammation and digestive issues.

What to Do

- Gradually reduce or eliminate irritants like:
  - Highly processed snacks and fast foods.
  - Sugary beverages or excessive caffeine.
  - Alcohol or artificial sweeteners like aspartame.

Elimination Diet: If you suspect specific foods are contributing to your symptoms, consider an elimination diet:

- Remove common triggers like gluten, dairy, soy, and nightshades for 2–4 weeks.
- Reintroduce these foods one at a time to identify any that exacerbate pain or digestive discomfort.

What About Lectins?

Lectins, found in foods like beans, lentils, and nightshades, can irritate the gut lining in sensitive individuals. If you notice symptoms after eating these foods, you might reduce or avoid them temporarily, but most people tolerate lectins well when foods are prepared properly (e.g., soaking beans or cooking thoroughly).

3. Repair Your Gut Lining

Why It Works

Your gut lining acts as a barrier, keeping harmful substances out of your bloodstream. Chronic pain and inflammation can weaken this barrier, leading to "leaky gut." Supporting gut repair strengthens this barrier, reduces inflammation, and improves resilience.

Long-term use of proton pump inhibitors (PPIs), often prescribed to manage acid reflux or counteract the effects of NSAIDs, can interfere with gut health by depleting critical nutrients and altering your gut's microbiome. While PPIs are helpful for short-term symptom relief, chronic use may contribute to issues like magnesium and vitamin B12 deficiency, poor calcium absorption (affecting bone health), and increased susceptibility to gut infections.

What to Do

- **If You Use PPIs**: Talk to your healthcare provider about testing for nutrient deficiencies and exploring whether it's possible to reduce your reliance on PPIs.
- **Alternatives to Consider**:
  - **Dietary Adjustments**: Avoid trigger foods like spicy or acidic items, and eat smaller, more frequent meals.
  - **Lifestyle Changes**: Elevate your head while sleeping and avoid lying down right after meals.
  - **Natural Options**: Digestive bitters or deglycyrrhizinated licorice (DGL) can soothe the gut lining and reduce reflux symptoms.

Gut-Healing Nutrients

- **L-Glutamine**: Found in bone broth, chicken, or supplements, it supports gut lining repair.
- **Zinc and Zinc Carnosine**: Zinc supports immune function and gut barrier health, while zinc carnosine specifically adheres to the gut lining to promote healing.
- **Collagen**: Found in bone broth or supplements, it provides structural support for the gut lining.

Advanced Option: Stool Testing

For persistent symptoms, stool testing can offer insights into your microbiome, inflammation levels, and digestive efficiency. Discuss this option with your healthcare provider to explore whether it might help guide your healing plan.

Pro Tip

If you're considering supplements like zinc carnosine or exploring alternatives to PPIs, consult your doctor for personalized advice.

"Could you add one gut-healing food, like bone broth or a zinc-rich meal, to your diet this week? Have you noticed how your diet or medications might influence your gut health?"

Restoring gut health is about more than improving digestion—it's about creating a foundation for resilience that influences every part of your body. By incorporating gut-friendly foods, repairing the gut lining, and minimizing irritants, you can begin to heal the gut-brain connection and reduce pain's grip on your life.

Start small, with one step or one habit at a time. Every choice you make to support your gut health is a step toward healing and thriving.

The gut isn't just connected to digestion—it also influences your sleep. Disruptions in gut health can affect melatonin production, a hormone critical for your sleep-wake cycle. By supporting your gut, you're also laying the groundwork for better, more restorative rest.

IMPROVING SLEEP TO ENHANCE RECOVERY

Sleep is one of the most powerful tools for healing and resilience. During deep sleep, your body carries out essential processes like repairing tissues, producing growth hormone, and regulating inflammation. But chronic pain often disrupts sleep, leading to a vicious cycle: poor sleep worsens pain, and pain makes it harder to sleep.

Good sleep hygiene—the practices and habits that promote restful sleep—can help you break this cycle. Improving your sleep isn't about perfection—it's about creating small, consistent habits that support better rest. This section focuses on actionable steps to restore your sleep patterns and enhance your body's recovery.

Key Actions to Improve Sleep Hygiene

1. Stick to a Consistent Sleep Schedule

Why It Works

Your body's internal clock, or circadian rhythm, thrives on consistency. Going to bed and waking up at the same time every day helps regulate melatonin production, improve sleep quality, and synchronize your body's healing processes.

What to Do

- Choose a consistent bedtime and wake-up time that works with your lifestyle, even on weekends.
- Create a calming pre-sleep routine, such as reading, meditating, or stretching, to signal to your body that it's time to wind down.

Pro Tip

Pair your bedtime routine with a relaxing scent like lavender or chamomile to condition your mind for sleep.

"What time do you usually go to bed? Could you try sticking to the same schedule for a week and see how it feels?"

---

2. Optimize Your Sleep Environment

Why It Works

A quiet, dark, and comfortable sleep environment reduces distractions and signals your brain that it's time to rest.

What to Do

- **Darkness**: Use blackout curtains or an eye mask to block light.
- **Noise**: Consider a white noise machine or earplugs to mask disruptive sounds.
- **Comfort**: Invest in a supportive mattress and breathable bedding.

Pro Tip

Keep your bedroom cool—around 65°F (18°C)—as lower temperatures encourage deeper sleep.

"Is there anything about your bedroom that might be affecting your sleep? How could you make it more restful?"

---

3. Limit Blue Light Exposure in the Evening

Why It Works

Blue light from screens (phones, tablets, TVs) interferes with melatonin production, making it harder for your body to transition into sleep mode.

What to Do

- Turn off screens at least 1 hour before bed.
- If you need to use screens, use blue-light-blocking glasses or apps like f.lux to reduce blue light exposure.

Pro Tip

Replace screen time with relaxing activities like journaling, reading a physical book, or practicing deep breathing.

"Could you try turning off screens earlier tonight? What relaxing activity could you do instead?"

---

4. Incorporate Relaxation Techniques Before Bed

Why It Works

Stress and tension make it harder to fall and stay asleep. Relaxation techniques calm the nervous system, making it easier to drift into restful sleep.

What to Do

- Practice 5–10 minutes of deep breathing, progressive muscle relaxation, or guided meditation before bed.
- Experiment with gentle yoga stretches to release physical tension.

Pro Tip

Apps like Calm or Insight Timer offer guided meditations specifically designed for sleep.

"What's one small way you could unwind before bed tonight? Could you try a relaxation exercise?"

5. Address Daytime Habits That Impact Sleep

Why It Works

Sleep isn't just about what happens at night—daytime habits like caffeine intake, exercise, and sunlight exposure influence your body's ability to sleep well.

What to Do

- **Caffeine**: Avoid caffeine after 2 p.m. to minimize its effects on sleep.
- **Exercise**: Incorporate regular movement but avoid intense workouts late in the evening.
- **Sunlight**: Get 10–15 minutes of morning sunlight to help regulate your circadian rhythm.

"Are there any daytime habits—like caffeine or screen time—that might be affecting your sleep? What's one small change you could try?"

Sleep isn't just a passive activity—it's an essential part of your body's recovery and resilience. By focusing on sleep hygiene, such as creating a consistent routine, optimizing your environment, and practicing relaxation techniques, you can set the stage for deeper, more restorative rest.

Start small. Even one change, like turning off screens earlier or adding a calming bedtime ritual, can make a difference. Over time, these habits will help you reclaim the healing power of sleep.

Sleep is one of the cornerstones of resilience, but it's just one piece of the puzzle. By combining better sleep hygiene with daily habits that support your nervous system, gut health, and energy, you can create a powerful routine for long-term recovery. In the next section, we'll explore how to weave these strategies into your daily life in a way that feels sustainable and empowering.

BUILDING BIOLOGICAL RESILIENCE AS A DAILY PRACTICE

Resilience isn't built in a day—it's a series of small, consistent actions that compound over time. Biological resilience involves creating habits that support your body's ability to heal, regulate itself, and adapt to challenges. This final section pulls together the strategies from this chapter and offers tools to help you integrate them into your daily life.

Building resilience is not about following a rigid routine—it's about discovering what works for you and adapting as you go. You might find that some strategies resonate immediately, while others take more time to integrate. The key is to start small, focus on what feels manageable, and allow yourself the freedom to adjust.

By focusing on consistency rather than perfection, you can make resilience a part of your routine, improving not only your recovery but also your overall quality of life.

Key Steps for Daily Biological Resilience

1. Start Small and Build Gradually

Why It Works

Big changes can feel overwhelming and unsustainable. Starting with one or two small habits makes it easier to stay consistent and build momentum.

What to Do

- Choose one or two strategies from this chapter to focus on first. For example:
  - Practice 5 minutes of deep breathing each morning.
  - Add one anti-inflammatory food to your meals daily.
  - Stick to a consistent bedtime for one week.

Pro Tip

Use a habit tracker or journal to celebrate your wins, no matter how small.

"What's one small habit you could start today to support your biological resilience?"

---

2. Use Tools to Track Progress

Why It Works

Tracking helps you stay accountable and provides tangible evidence of your growth, which can be motivating during challenging times.

What to Do

- Use a journal, app, or checklist to track your daily habits.
- Record how you feel physically and emotionally as you build new habits.

Tech Options

- There are several great apps for tracking habits.
- Smart devices like hydration-tracking water bottles or fitness trackers for movement and sleep.

"Could you try tracking one habit this week? What would you like to measure?"

There's no one right way to build resilience. Tracking tools like apps or journals are there to support you, but if a structured approach doesn't feel right for you, that's okay. You can reflect informally—jotting down a thought in a notebook or simply noticing what's working in your day.

3. Prioritize Recovery and Rest

Why It Works

Resilience doesn't mean pushing through exhaustion—it's about knowing when to rest so your body can repair and recharge.

What to Do

- Schedule breaks during your day to avoid burnout.
- Take rest days from physical activity when needed, focusing on gentle movement like stretching or a short walk.

Pro Tip

Build rest into your weekly routine—think of it as an investment in your resilience.

> *"When was the last time you truly rested? How can you create space for rest this week?"*

4. Reflect and Adjust Over Time

Why It Works

Resilience isn't a one-size-fits-all journey. Reflecting on what's working (and what isn't) helps you make adjustments that align with your needs and goals.

What to Do

- Set aside 5–10 minutes weekly to review your progress. Ask yourself:
    - What went well this week?
    - What challenges did I face?
    - How can I adjust my approach for next week?

Pro Tip

Be kind to yourself—progress isn't always linear, but every step forward counts.

"What's one thing you're proud of this week? How can you build on that success?"

Building biological resilience is a journey, not a sprint. Each small habit you practice—whether it's eating anti-inflammatory foods, improving your sleep hygiene, or simply pausing to breathe—strengthens your foundation for healing.

You don't need to do everything at once. Start with one change, track your progress, and celebrate your wins. Over time, these habits will become part of your daily life, helping you thrive beyond pain.

TURNING RESILIENCE INTO A WAY OF LIFE

In this chapter, you've explored how to rebuild your body's biological resilience—calming your nervous system, reducing inflammation, repairing cellular health, and restoring balance to your gut and hormones. These are powerful tools, not just for managing chronic pain, but for creating a foundation of strength, energy, and healing.

Resilience doesn't come from drastic overhauls or fleeting changes. It's built from the small, consistent steps you take every day. Whether you're practicing deep breathing, swapping in anti-inflammatory foods, or committing to a better sleep routine, each choice strengthens your body's ability to adapt and thrive.

Imagine waking up with more energy, feeling your body work for you instead of against you. What's one small step you can take today to begin turning that vision into reality?

Biological resilience is just one piece of the puzzle. Chronic pain isn't just about what's happening in your body—it's also deeply connected to the way your mind processes stress, emotions, and pain signals.

In the next chapter, we'll explore psychological resilience—how to rewire your brain, manage stress, and build the mental strength to regain focus and joy in your life. Together, these tools will help you reclaim your life from pain and reconnect with what truly matters.

CHAPTER 14
REBUILDING AND AMPLIFYING PSYCHOLOGICAL RESILIENCE

Chronic pain doesn't just affect your body—it reshapes your brain. Pain pathways in the nervous system become overactive, stress amplifies the experience of discomfort, and negative thought patterns take root, creating a loop that feels impossible to escape. This isn't "all in your head"; it's a real, physiological response to living with persistent pain.

Just as physical therapy helps restore strength and mobility to injured muscles, building psychological resilience helps heal the parts of your brain affected by chronic pain. This process is backed by science: the brain is remarkably adaptable through a process called neuroplasticity. With the right practices, you can unlearn pain-amplifying patterns and create new ones that promote calm, clarity, and resilience.

We know this isn't the first time you've encountered the idea of addressing the psychological aspect of pain in this book. That repetition is intentional. Many people hesitate to embrace the psychological component of pain recovery, believing that pain is solely a physical issue. It's a common and understandable reaction, but embracing this truth is essential to your healing journey.

Psychological resilience isn't about ignoring your pain or pretending it's not real—it's about working with your brain, just as you work with your body in physical therapy. Pain is a whole-body experience, shaped by the ways your brain interprets signals from your body. By strengthening your mind's ability to adapt, you're giving yourself a critical tool to reduce pain's intensity and reclaim your life.

Think of it this way: if a smoke alarm in your home goes off, it's a vital signal that something might be wrong. But sometimes, smoke alarms become too sensitive, blaring loudly at the slightest hint of toast burning. Chronic pain works in a similar way—your nervous system becomes hypersensitive, sending pain signals even when there's no true danger. By rewiring how your brain interprets these signals, you can help "reset" the alarm, reducing pain's grip.

SETTING THE STAGE FOR WHAT'S AHEAD

In this chapter, we'll explore practical ways to build psychological resilience. You'll learn how to:

Recognize and reframe unhelpful thought patterns that amplify pain.

Break the pain-stress cycle by managing your emotional and physiological responses.

Harness the power of neuroplasticity to train your brain toward calm and control.

Focus on your personal mission to shift your attention away from pain and toward what truly matters.

These strategies aren't about dismissing your pain—they're about helping you respond to it in new, empowering ways. Just as small steps in physical therapy rebuild strength over time, each mental shift strengthens your brain's capacity to adapt and thrive.

> **Key Takeaways:**
> **Building Psychological Resilience**
> Practices like mindfulness and reframing help break these loops, reducing stress and fear. Small, consistent changes retrain the brain for resilience and calm.

THE POWER OF PERSPECTIVE

Your thoughts shape your reality, and this is especially true when it comes to chronic pain. Pain isn't just a physical sensation—it's deeply tied to how your brain processes stress and emotions. When you're living with pain, unhelpful thought patterns like fear or catastrophizing don't just feel overwhelming—they actually strengthen the neural pathways associated with pain, amplifying its intensity.

But here's the good news: your brain is always learning. Every thought, feeling, and behavior trains your brain in one direction or another. If you consistently think, "This pain will never improve," your brain becomes better at reinforcing that belief. But if you train your brain to recognize possibility and resilience, it will adapt in ways that reduce pain's hold on your life.

We're not diving into these ideas just for the sake of science. Chronic pain is as much a physical issue as it is a psychological one—and the treatments we're discussing have very real, physical effects on your brain. The tools you're about to learn aren't abstract or theoretical—they're rooted in your brain's natural ability to heal and adapt.

KEY CONCEPT: COGNITIVE DISTORTIONS, THE BRAIN, AND CHRONIC PAIN

Negative thought patterns like catastrophizing activate the default mode network (DMN) in your brain—a network that becomes hyperactive in people with chronic pain. The DMN is responsible for ruminating on past experiences and anticipating future problems, which can make pain feel inescapable.

Chronic pain also affects the anterior cingulate cortex (ACC) and prefrontal cortex (PFC)—areas responsible for emotional regulation and decision-making. These changes are physical and measurable, and they make it harder to break free from negative thought patterns.

The strategies in this section are designed to reverse these changes. By intentionally practicing tools like reframing thoughts or visualizing calm, you're training the ACC and PFC to regain control while quieting the DMN. These aren't just mental exercises—they're ways to physically rewire your brain for resilience.

Actionable Strategies

1. **Identify Your Thought Patterns**

Why It Works

Awareness of your thoughts helps you interrupt automatic reactions that perpetuate pain. Research shows that simply observing negative thought patterns activates the prefrontal cort**ex**, which helps regulate the emotional response to pain.

What to Do

- Keep a thought journal for a few days. Whenever pain feels overwhelming, write down:
    - The situation or trigger (e.g., "I missed work because of pain").
    - The automatic thoughts you had (e.g., "I'm letting everyone down").
    - How those thoughts made you feel emotionally and physically.

- Look for patterns. Are certain distortions, like catastrophizing or all-or-nothing thinking, showing up repeatedly?

___

"What's one recurring thought about your pain that you'd like to challenge?"

___

2. Reframe Unhelpful Thoughts

Why It Works

Reframing engages the prefrontal cortex and anterior cingulate cortex, training these regions to regulate the brain's response to pain signals more effectively. Studies show that cognitive reframing can lower activity in the amygdala, the brain's fear center, reducing the emotional intensity of pain.

What to Do

- Use the "Cognitive Reframe" technique:
  1. Identify the unhelpful thought (e.g., "I'll never get better").
  2. Challenge it with evidence (e.g., "There are days when I feel better than others, so improvement is possible").
  3. Replace it with a balanced thought (e.g., "Healing is a process, and I'm taking steps to improve").
- Practice reframing one thought each day to build the habit.

Pro Tip

Use a reminder like a sticky note or phone alarm with a message like "Pause and reframe" to catch unhelpful thoughts in the moment.

> *"Can you think of a recent negative thought about pain? How could you reframe it in a way that feels more balanced?"*

3. Develop a "Pain Partner" Mindset

Why It Works

Shifting your emotional response to pain reduces its impact on the brain's pain-processing regions, including the somatosensory cortex. Visualizing pain as a misguided helper helps calm the insula, a brain region involved in the emotional experience of pain and increases parasympathetic (relaxation) activity.

Think back to Andre, who had spent years viewing his pain as an enemy that ended his soccer career. With practice, he began imagining his pain as a protective alarm that had become oversensitive. On a particularly painful day, instead of reacting with anger, he visualized thanking his pain for "trying to help" while calmly telling it, "I've got this under control." Over time, this mindset shift helped Andre feel less consumed by his pain, even on tough days.

What to Do

- When you feel pain, visualize it as a small child or a well-meaning but misguided friend who doesn't know how to help.
- Instead of reacting with frustration, imagine calmly explaining: "Thank you for trying to protect me, but I'm okay. I don't need this alarm right now."

Practical Tool

Write out your "pain partner" dialogue on a sticky note or journal. Keep it somewhere visible so you can remind yourself of this mindset during difficult moments.

What would your pain say to you if it could talk? How might you respond with compassion?

Every thought you have is part of a feedback loop. You're always training your brain—so why not train it to work in your favor? By learning to recognize and reframe unhelpful patterns, you're creating new neural pathways that reduce pain's intensity and control.

You might be skeptical of how much this can help, but remember: these changes are real, physical, and grounded in your brain's natural ability to adapt. The process takes time, but each small shift makes resilience easier and more automatic.

BREAKING THE PAIN-STRESS CYCLE

What Happens in a Stress Response

When your brain detects a threat—whether it's a real danger or persistent pain—it activates your stress response. This automatic reaction, controlled by the hypothalamic-pituitary-adrenal (HPA) axis and the sympathetic nervous system (SNS), is designed to keep you safe in the short term.

Here's what happens physiologically:

- **Cortisol and Adrenaline Surge**: Your adrenal glands flood your body with hormones, increasing heart rate, raising blood pressure, and delivering extra glucose to your muscles.

- **Shallow, Rapid Breathing**: The SNS triggers shallow breathing to increase oxygen intake quickly. However, over time, this can disrupt CO_2 levels, leading to symptoms like dizziness, muscle tension, and anxiety.
- **Pain Amplification**: Stress makes the brain's pain-processing regions, including the insula and anterior cingulate cortex (ACC), more active, amplifying discomfort.

Pain and stress share overlapping pathways in the brain. When pain becomes chronic, this stress response can stay "on" even when no real threat exists. Over time, this feedback loop rewires your brain to prioritize pain signals, making the experience feel more intense.

Why It Matters

Breaking this cycle isn't just about "relaxing"—it's about rewiring your brain to de-escalate the stress response, reducing both the perception and impact of pain. The good news? By retraining your body's breathing patterns and calming your nervous system, you can break this loop and create a foundation for healing.

Key Techniques to Break the Stress Response

1. **Diaphragmatic Breathing and CO2 Tolerance**

Why It Works

Shallow breathing disrupts your body's CO_2 balance, which can trigger or worsen anxiety. Diaphragmatic breathing retrains your body to tolerate normal CO_2 levels, reducing the hyperventilation cycle and calming your nervous system. It also helps activate the parasympathetic nervous system, which reduces the stress response.

What to Do

We've already discussed how to practice diaphragmatic breathing in chapter twelve, focusing on its physical benefits. If you need a refresher, revisit that section for detailed instructions.

Here, it's worth noting that diaphragmatic breathing also has a significant psychological role. By slowing your breath and extending your exhale, you send a signal to your brain that it's safe to relax, reducing anxiety and calming overactive pain signals.

"When could you take a few minutes today to practice this simple breathing technique and notice its calming effect?"

---

2. Mindful Meditation

Why It Works

Mindfulness trains your brain to observe pain and stress without judgment, helping you detach from unhelpful mental patterns. This can weaken pain pathways in the brain and reduce activity in the default mode network (DMN), which is responsible for overthinking and rumination.

What to Do

1. Find a comfortable, quiet place to sit or lie down.
2. Close your eyes and bring your attention to your breath or a simple focal point, like the feeling of your hands resting on your lap.
3. When your mind wanders (and it will), gently bring your focus back to your breath.

4. Start with 5 minutes, gradually increasing to 10–20 minutes as it feels comfortable.

Dispelling the "Active Mind" Myth

You might think, "I can't meditate—my mind is too busy." That's actually the point. Meditation isn't about stopping your thoughts—it's about noticing them without following every trail they create. Over time, this helps you build the skill of letting go, which reduces stress and rumination.

Pro Tip

Use a guided meditation app like Calm or Insight Timer if you're unsure how to begin.

"What's one part of your day when you could set aside 5 minutes for mindfulness?"

---

3. Heart Coherence Techniques

What Is Heart Coherence?

Heart coherence is the state of achieving smooth, balanced heart rhythms, which calms the nervous system and improves communication between the heart and brain. By focusing on positive emotions and rhythmic breathing, you can shift your body from stress (sympathetic dominance) to relaxation (parasympathetic activation).

How to Practice It

1. **Focus on the Heart**: Sit comfortably and place your hand over your heart. Imagine your breath flowing in and out of your chest area.
2. **Activate Positive Emotion**: Think of a memory or feeling that brings you joy, gratitude, or calm—like a loved one's smile or a moment in nature. Hold onto that emotion.
3. **Maintain the Connection**: Breathe in a steady rhythm (e.g., 5 seconds in, 5 seconds out) for 3–5 minutes.

Why It Works

Heart coherence increases heart rate variability (HRV), which measures the flexibility of your nervous system. Think of HRV as a sign of how well your body can shift between stress and relaxation. Higher HRV means your body is more adaptable, promoting resilience and emotional balance.

Why It Matters

Studies show that practicing heart coherence not only lowers stress but also strengthens communication between the heart and brain. This connection helps calm the amygdala (the brain's alarm system), reducing emotional reactivity and physical tension.

Pro Tip

Devices like HeartMath's Inner Balance tracker can provide real-time feedback on your HRV, helping you track progress and deepen your practice.

"What's one memory or thought that consistently brings you joy or calm? Could you use it to practice heart coherence today?"

SCIENCE SPOTLIGHT

Each of these techniques targets the brain and body systems involved in stress:

- **Diaphragmatic Breathing** recalibrates CO_2 levels and stimulates the Vagus nerve to reduce SNS dominance.
- **Mindfulness Meditation** reduces DMN activity and increases prefrontal cortex regulation, improving your brain's ability to manage pain and stress.
- **Heart Coherence** balances HRV and strengthens the heart-brain connection, creating a powerful state of calm and focus.

Breaking the pain-stress cycle isn't about perfection—it's about creating small, manageable moments of calm. Each time you practice diaphragmatic breathing, mindfulness, or heart coherence, you're teaching your body and brain to work together, reducing pain's grip and restoring balance.

Which of these tools will you try today? Even one small step can create a ripple effect, helping you reclaim control over your stress response and your life.

Breaking the pain-stress cycle is the first step in rewiring your brain. When you calm your body's stress response, you create the foundation for neuroplasticity—the brain's ability to form new, healthier pathways. In the next section, we'll explore how intentional practices like visualization and gratitude can actively reshape your brain to reduce pain and build resilience.

HARNESSING NEUROPLASTICITY TO REWIRE THE BRAIN

THE BRAIN'S AMAZING ABILITY TO CHANGE

Chronic pain rewires the brain. Over time, pain strengthens neural pathways associated with discomfort and stress, making the brain more sensitive to pain signals. This doesn't mean your pain isn't real—it means your brain has adapted to prioritize pain, like a broken record that repeats the same message.

The good news? Your brain is capable of neuroplasticity—the ability to reorganize and form new connections. Just as chronic pain rewires the brain in unhelpful ways, you can train it to create new, healthier patterns that reduce pain sensitivity and improve emotional balance.

Think of it like a well-worn hiking trail. Pain has created a deep rut that your brain automatically follows. But with practice, you can carve out a new path—one that prioritizes calm, resilience, and healing.

KEY CONCEPT: HOW NEUROPLASTICITY WORKS

Neuroplasticity is the brain's ability to change in response to new experiences, thoughts, and behaviors. It's a process of "use it or lose it":

- **Use it**: Repeating helpful thoughts or actions strengthens the neural connections that support them, making them easier and more automatic.
- **Lose it**: When unhelpful patterns, like rumination or catastrophizing, aren't used as often, the brain weakens those pathways over time.

In chronic pain, the pain matrix—a network involving the somatosensory cortex, insula, and anterior cingulate cortex (ACC)—becomes overactive. By intentionally practicing techniques that focus on calm and control, you can quiet the pain matrix and strengthen areas like the prefrontal cortex, which helps regulate emotions and attention.

Actionable Strategies

1. **Visualization and Guided Imagery**

Why It Works

Visualization activates the same neural pathways as physical actions, helping the brain "practice" new responses to pain without reinforcing the old ones. Research shows that guided imagery can reduce pain intensity and increase relaxation by altering activity in the pain matrix.

What to Do

1. Find a quiet, comfortable place to sit or lie down.
2. Close your eyes and imagine a scene that makes you feel safe, calm, or joyful—like a beach, a forest, or a favorite memory.
3. Engage all your senses. For example:
    - See the soft waves or vibrant greenery.
    - Hear the gentle rustle of leaves or the rhythm of the ocean.
    - Feel the warmth of the sun on your skin or the cool breeze.
4. Spend 5–10 minutes in this scene, focusing on the sensations and emotions it evokes.

Pro Tip

For pain-specific visualization, imagine the pain as a physical object (like a knot or a block of ice) that melts or dissolves with each exhale.

"What's one calming or joyful memory you could use as the focus for your visualization?"

2. Mental Rehearsal for Resilience

Why It Works

Mental rehearsal strengthens the neural pathways associated with resilience and coping, much like how athletes use visualization to improve performance. By imagining yourself navigating pain with calm and confidence, you're training your brain to respond that way in real life.

What to Do

1. Close your eyes and picture yourself in a situation where pain might normally feel overwhelming—like walking up stairs or attending a social event.
2. Imagine yourself moving through the experience with ease, confidence, and calm.
3. Focus on how it feels to succeed—strong, capable, and in control.

Pro Tip

Pair this with affirmations like, "I can handle this," or "My body and mind are strong."

"What's one situation you could mentally rehearse this week to build confidence in managing pain?"

3. Gratitude Practices

Why It Works

Gratitude shifts your brain's focus from stress and pain to positive experiences. Neuroscience research shows that gratitude increases activity in the prefrontal cortex, which enhances emotional regulation, and decreases activity in the amygdala, reducing fear and stress responses.

Why It Matters

Regular gratitude practice can also boost levels of serotonin and dopamine—chemicals that promote feelings of well-being—creating long-term changes in how your brain processes positive and negative experiences.

When to Practice

- **Morning Gratitude**: Sets a positive tone for the day, framing your mindset around abundance and possibility.
- **Evening Gratitude**: Helps you reflect on the positives of the day, reducing stress and improving sleep quality.

You can try either or both, depending on what fits your schedule and needs.

What to Do

1. At the end of each day, write down 3 things you're grateful for.
2. They can be big or small—like a kind word from a friend or a moment of sunshine.
3. Reflect on why these things matter to you and how they made you feel.

Practical Tool

Consider using a gratitude-specific journal, like the Five Minute Journal, or apps like Grateful or Gratitude Journal, which can send reminders to help you stay consistent.

Adaptability

If you're short on time, mentally list your gratitude items while brushing your teeth or preparing for bed.

Deepening the Practice

Feel gratitude in your body. As you reflect, notice any sensations that arise—warmth in your chest, a softening in your shoulders, or a sense of lightness. Breathe into these sensations, letting them expand with each inhale.

Pro Tip

If journaling feels overwhelming, mentally list your gratitude items during a walk or before bed.

"What's one thing you're grateful for right now, and where do you feel that gratitude in your body?"

SCIENCE SPOTLIGHT: HOW THESE PRACTICES REWIRE THE BRAIN

- **Visualization and Mental Rehearsal**: Activate the **motor cortex** and strengthen the connection between the prefrontal cortex and pain-processing regions, helping the brain learn new responses to pain.
- **Gratitude Practices**: Increase levels of serotonin and dopamine, the brain's "feel-good" chemicals, while reducing cortisol levels and stress.
- **Neuroplasticity as a Whole**: Over time, these practices weaken the brain's pain pathways and reinforce circuits that promote resilience and well-being.

Your brain is constantly learning. Each time you visualize calm, mentally rehearse confidence, or practice gratitude, you're training your brain to respond differently to pain. These small, intentional moments build up over time, creating new pathways for resilience and healing.

Imagine what it would feel like to navigate pain with calm and control. What's one small practice you can start today to begin carving that new path?

As you practice tools like visualization and gratitude, you're not just rewiring your brain—you're also strengthening your ability to manage emotions. Emotional regulation is a key part of resilience because pain doesn't just affect your body—it impacts your feelings and reactions. Let's explore how to regain control over your emotional responses and reduce pain's grip on your mind.

BUILDING EMOTIONAL REGULATION SKILLS

Living with chronic pain doesn't just affect your body—it challenges your emotions. Pain can bring frustration, sadness, anger, or hopelessness, and over time, these feelings can become overwhelming. Emotional responses don't just reflect how you feel; they actively influence your brain and body, amplifying the pain-stress cycle.

Imagine those rutted hiking paths in your brain again. Emotional reactions like fear or frustration deepen the rut, making it easier for your brain to default to those patterns. Emotional regulation is about carving out new trails—ones that lead to calm, balance, and resilience. By practicing these skills, you can teach your brain to respond differently, creating new pathways that weaken pain's grip and strengthen your ability to cope.

KEY CONCEPT: THE EMOTIONAL BRAIN IN CHRONIC PAIN

Chronic pain rewires the emotional brain, particularly the amygdala, which becomes hyperactive. This can lead to what's known as an amygdala hijack—a state where fear, frustration, or anger take over, bypassing your brain's ability to think calmly and rationally.

During an amygdala hijack, the prefrontal cortex (the part of your brain responsible for decision-making and regulation) is essentially "shut out" of the process. This is why emotions can feel so overwhelming and why it's hard to think clearly during moments of distress.

Practicing emotional regulation teaches your brain to stay calm and engaged, even when the amygdala sends distress signals. Over time, these practices strengthen the prefrontal cortex, reducing the intensity and frequency of amygdala hijacks.

Actionable Strategies

1. Self-Compassion Exercises

Why It Works

Practicing self-compassion interrupts the amygdala hijack, helping to calm your stress response. It activates the parasympathetic nervous system, which signals safety to your brain and body. It also reinforces the brain's caregiving system, reducing cortisol and increasing oxytocin (the bonding hormone).

Take Sarah, for example. After years of criticizing herself for not "pushing through" her pain, she started practicing self-compassion. On difficult days, instead of saying, "Why can't I just get over this?" she reminded herself, "This is a tough moment, and I'm doing the best I can." Over time, Sarah noticed she felt calmer and less emotionally exhausted, even on days when her pain didn't change.

What to Do

- **Acknowledge Your Struggle**: When you feel overwhelmed, say to yourself, "This is a tough moment. It's okay to feel this way."
- **Offer Yourself Kindness**: Imagine what you'd say to a close friend in your situation. Say those same words to yourself.
- **Practice Physical Soothing**: Place a hand on your heart or gently hug yourself as you take slow, deep breaths.

Pro Tip

Use phrases like, "I'm doing the best I can," or, "It's okay to not be okay right now," to remind yourself of your humanity.

"How can you show yourself kindness during moments of pain or frustration today?"

2. Journaling to Process Emotions

Why It Works

Writing about your emotions activates the prefrontal cortex, the part of your brain responsible for emotional regulation and decision-making. Studies show that journaling helps reduce activity in the amygdala, your brain's fear center, which can lower the intensity of negative emotions and improve your ability to cope with stress.

For example, Michael struggled with feelings of anger and frustration over how pain had changed his life. When he started journaling, he wrote about these emotions freely, not worrying about grammar or structure. Over time, he began to notice patterns—like how frustration often arose after pushing himself too hard. Journaling helped Michael process his feelings and gave him insights into what he could adjust in his day-to-day life.

What to Do

1. Spend 5–10 minutes writing about how you feel, without worrying about grammar or structure.
2. Reflect on these questions:
    - What emotions am I feeling right now?
    - What might have triggered these feelings?
    - What's one small step I could take to feel more balanced?

Practical Tool

If writing feels overwhelming, try using a journaling app like Day One or Journey, which offer prompts to guide your reflections. Alternatively, use voice memos to record your thoughts when journaling by hand feels difficult.

> *"When you're feeling overwhelmed, could journaling help you process and release those emotions?"*

3. Creating Emotional Anchors

Why It Works

Emotional anchors are tools or rituals that ground you when emotions feel overwhelming. They help redirect attention and calm the amygdala, creating space for emotional regulation. Anchors provide a tangible way to step back from distress and connect with a sense of calm and safety.

What to Do

Choose an anchor that feels comforting, such as:

- A favorite song or playlist.
- A small object, like a stone or charm, that you can hold in your hand.
- A soothing scent, like lavender or eucalyptus.

Use your anchor during moments of distress. Focus on how it feels, smells, or sounds, allowing it to bring you back to the present.

Pro Tip

Over time, your brain will associate your anchor with calm, making it more effective with practice.

"What's one object, song, or ritual that helps you feel calm and grounded?"

SCIENCE SPOTLIGHT: THE NEUROSCIENCE OF EMOTIONAL REGULATION

- **Amygdala Hijack**: Emotional regulation skills like self-compassion and journaling help re-engage the prefrontal cortex during an amygdala hijack, allowing you to respond to emotions thoughtfully rather than react impulsively.
- **Self-Compassion**: Activates the brain's caregiving system, increasing oxytocin and reducing cortisol.
- **Journaling**: Reduces amygdala activity, helping the brain process emotions without becoming overwhelmed.
- **Anchors**: Strengthen the brain's connection to soothing experiences, creating a shortcut to emotional balance.

Emotions are powerful, but they don't have to control you. Each time you practice self-compassion, journal your feelings, or use an emotional anchor, you're teaching your brain new ways to respond to pain and stress.

Imagine navigating pain with less frustration and more calm. What's one small emotional regulation skill you can try today to take that first step?

Emotional regulation helps you find balance in the moment, but resilience also requires a deeper sense of purpose. Pain often narrows your world, making it hard to focus on what matters most. Reconnecting with your personal mission gives you a powerful reason to move forward and helps you reshape your life around meaning, not just pain.

STRENGTHENING FOCUS ON YOUR PERSONAL MISSION: RECLAIMING WHAT MATTERS MOST

Chronic pain has a way of narrowing your world. Over time, it can overshadow your goals, relationships, and sense of purpose, making life feel smaller and more constrained. It's easy to feel like your pain defines you or to lose sight of what truly matters most.

But focusing on a personal mission—a deep sense of purpose that aligns with your values and passions—can help you widen your perspective again. When you reconnect with what matters, you shift your brain's attention away from pain and toward meaningful, fulfilling goals.

Building focus on your mission isn't about ignoring your pain—it's about redefining how much space it takes up in your life. By strengthening this focus, you carve a new path in your brain that prioritizes hope, action, and resilience.

KEY CONCEPT: PURPOSE AS A PAIN BUFFER

Research shows that having a sense of purpose can reduce the brain's sensitivity to pain. When you're engaged in meaningful activities, areas of the brain associated with focus and reward—like the prefrontal cortex and the ventral striatum—become more active. This activity quiets the pain-processing regions, such as the insula and somatosensory cortex, effectively reducing pain's impact.

Purpose also acts as a buffer against stress, increasing resilience and emotional regulation. Reconnecting with your mission gives you a powerful reason to move forward, even on the hardest days.

Actionable Strategies

1. Reflect on Your "Why"

Why It Works

Reconnecting with your core values and passions shifts your focus from what pain has taken to what still drives you. It helps you create a mental anchor that keeps you grounded during challenging moments.

What to Do

1. Set aside 10–15 minutes to reflect on the following questions:
    - What activities or experiences make me feel alive or fulfilled?
    - Who or what inspires me to keep going, even when it's hard?
    - What are three things I value most in life?
2. Write your responses down in a journal or notebook. Let them serve as a personal reminder of your mission when pain feels overwhelming.

Pro Tip

If journaling feels difficult, try voice-recording your reflections or creating a vision board with images that represent your purpose.

"What's one thing that brings meaning to your life, no matter how small?"

---

2. Set Mission-Focused Goals

Why It Works

Focusing on small, meaningful goals shifts your attention away from pain and toward what matters most. It reinforces pathways in the brain associated with motivation and reward, creating positive feedback loops.

What to Do

1. Choose one goal that aligns with your mission—something that feels important, even if it's small.
   - Example: If your mission involves supporting your family, your goal could be to spend 10 minutes of quality time with them today.
   - Example: If your mission is rooted in creativity, your goal might be to sketch or write for 5 minutes.
2. Break the goal into manageable steps, making it realistic and achievable.

Pro Tip

Use the SMART framework to guide your goals:

- **Specific**: Be clear about what you want to achieve.
- **Measurable**: Track your progress.
- **Achievable**: Set a goal that feels doable.
- **Relevant**: Align it with your mission.
- **Time-bound**: Set a deadline or timeframe.

"What's one small step you could take this week toward a goal that aligns with your mission?"

---

3. Use Gratitude to Reinforce Your Mission

Why It Works

Gratitude deepens your connection to the people, activities, and values that matter most. It strengthens the brain's reward pathways, creating a sense of fulfillment and reinforcing your focus on your mission.

What to Do

1. Each day, reflect on one thing related to your mission that you're grateful for. For example:
   - "I'm grateful for the chance to support my family today."
   - "I'm grateful for the creativity I expressed in my painting."
2. Pair this gratitude with a physical sensation—like a deep breath or placing your hand on your chest—to deepen its impact.

Pro Tip

Keep a small object, like a bracelet or stone, as a physical reminder of your mission. Each time you see or hold it, reflect on what you're grateful for.

"What's one part of your mission that you can feel gratitude for today?"

SCIENCE SPOTLIGHT: THE POWER OF PURPOSE

- **Brain Changes**: Purpose increases activity in the **prefrontal cortex**, which improves focus and emotional regulation. It also quiets pain-processing regions like the **insula** and **somatosensory cortex**, reducing the intensity of pain.
- **Stress Buffering**: A strong sense of purpose reduces cortisol levels and increases heart rate variability (HRV), both markers of improved resilience.
- **Motivation and Reward**: Engaging with meaningful goals activates the brain's reward system, creating positive feedback loops that sustain motivation.

Reconnecting with your mission is one of the most powerful steps you can take toward resilience. Each time you reflect on your "why," set a meaningful goal, or express gratitude for what matters most, you're shifting your brain's focus from pain to purpose.

What's one small step you can take today to strengthen your connection to your mission? Whether it's reflecting on your values, pursuing a goal, or simply noticing what brings you joy, each action reinforces your path to resilience.

BUILDING PSYCHOLOGICAL RESILIENCE AS A DAILY PRACTICE: SMALL STEPS, BIG CHANGES

Resilience isn't built in a single day—it's a skill developed through small, consistent actions. Just like exercising a muscle, the more you practice psychological resilience, the stronger it becomes. Over time, these daily habits can reshape your brain, quiet pain pathways, and empower you to live with greater calm, focus, and control.

This section ties together everything you've learned in this chapter, showing how to integrate these tools into your daily life. By creating a personalized routine and tracking your progress, you can build momentum, celebrate small wins, and keep moving forward—even when the journey feels challenging.

KEY CONCEPT: THE POWER OF CONSISTENCY

Neuroplasticity thrives on repetition. Every time you practice mindfulness, reframe a negative thought, or focus on your personal mission, you're strengthening the neural pathways that support resilience. Consistency is key—small, intentional steps practiced regularly are far more effective than occasional big efforts.

Actionable Strategies

1. **Create a Resilience Routine**

Why It Works

A daily routine makes resilience-building automatic, reducing the mental effort required to practice these skills. It also helps reinforce positive habits, creating a sense of structure and stability.

What to Do

1. Choose 2–3 practices from this chapter to include in your daily routine, such as:
    - 5 minutes of mindful meditation in the morning.
    - A gratitude reflection at the end of the day.
    - Journaling your emotions or setting a mission-focused goal.
2. Schedule these practices into your day, pairing them with existing habits (e.g., journaling after your morning coffee or meditating before bed).

Practical Tool

Use a habit-tracking app like Habitica, Streaks, or Way of Life to track these practices and celebrate your consistency. For paper-based options, try a daily planner or bullet journal to log your resilience-building habits.

The Ripple Effect

Small, consistent practices may seem insignificant at first, but over time, they create ripples of positive change throughout your life. For example:

- A single moment of mindfulness might help you feel calmer during a flare-up, which leads to better communication with loved ones or more restful sleep.
- Reflecting on gratitude can shift your perspective, making you more optimistic and less reactive to stress.

These ripples extend outward, affecting not just your mental state but your physical resilience, relationships, and overall sense of well-being.

Pro Tip

Start small. Focus on consistency rather than perfection—missing a day doesn't mean starting over, just continuing.

"What's one small resilience practice you could start building into your daily routine today, knowing it could create ripples of positive change?"

---

2. Track Your Progress

Why It Works

Tracking helps you stay accountable and motivated. It also lets you see how far you've come, even when progress feels slow.

What to Do

1. Use a journal, app, or simple checklist to track your resilience practices.
2. At the end of each week, reflect on:
   - What went well?
   - What felt challenging?
   - What's one adjustment you can make for next week?

Pro Tip

Celebrate small wins, like completing a week of consistent practices or noticing a positive change in your mood or outlook.

"How could tracking your progress help you stay consistent and motivated?"

---

3. Be Flexible and Adapt Over Time

Why It Works

Your needs and goals may shift over time, and your resilience practices should evolve with them. Flexibility helps you stay engaged and ensures that your routine continues to meet your needs.

What to Do

1. Revisit your routine every few weeks or months. Ask yourself:
   - What's working well?
   - What's no longer serving me?
   - What new practice could I try?
2. Adjust your routine to reflect your current priorities and challenges.

The Ripple Effect

Adjusting your practices doesn't erase your progress—it adds new ripples to your resilience journey. Each time you try something new or refine your habits, you're creating fresh pathways in your brain that expand your capacity to adapt and thrive.

Pro Tip

Be kind to yourself during setbacks. Progress isn't linear, and resilience is about continuing to show up, even when it's hard.

"What's one way you could adjust your practices to better meet your needs right now, knowing each change creates new ripples of resilience?"

SCIENCE SPOTLIGHT: HOW DAILY PRACTICES BUILD RESILIENCE

- **Repetition and Neuroplasticity**: Repeated actions strengthen the brain's ability to form new, healthier pathways, reducing the dominance of pain-related circuits.
- **Habit Formation**: Regular practices rewire the brain's

reward system, making positive behaviors more automatic over time.
- **Flexibility and Growth**: Adjusting your routine in response to challenges strengthens the brain's adaptability, a key component of resilience.

Andre's Journey to Building Resilience

For Andre, like many of our patients, mornings were the hardest—he dreaded getting out of bed, knowing his pain would follow her throughout the day. He often felt frustrated and overwhelmed, stuck in a cycle of negativity and exhaustion.

Andre decided to start small, choosing an effective three-practice plan.

1. **Morning Gratitude**: Each morning, he wrote down one thing she was grateful for, like a kind message from a student or a sunny day.
2. **Mindful Breathing**: Before bed, he practiced 5 minutes of diaphragmatic breathing to calm her racing thoughts.
3. **Mission-Focused Goals**: He set a goal to reconnect with her love of art by sketching for just 10 minutes twice a week.

At first, these changes seemed insignificant, but over time, Andre began to notice subtle shifts. The gratitude practice made his mornings feel lighter. Breathing exercises helped his fall asleep more easily, and the simple act of sketching brought his joy and a sense of accomplishment.

The ripple effect was undeniable: Andre's pain didn't disappear, but his mindset shifted. He felt calmer, more in control, and more connected to his sense of purpose. These small wins motivated him to keep going, eventually building a routine that transformed how he navigated his pain.

Affirmation: *I have the strength to rewire my mind, one small step at a time. My resilience grows with each practice.*

Psychological resilience is a journey of rewiring your brain, calming your emotions, and reconnecting with your purpose. Each small step—whether it's a moment of mindfulness, an act of self-compassion, or a gratitude practice—creates ripples of change that reshape your experience of pain. These ripples don't just affect your mind—they strengthen the foundation for biological and social resilience, too.

Psychological resilience is one pillar of your Peak Resilience Method, but it's deeply interconnected with the others. In the next chapter, we'll explore how social resilience—rebuilding and strengthening your relationships—can create a vital support system and can amplify these ripples pushing you forward on your healing journey.

CHAPTER 15
REBUILDING AND AMPLIFYING SOCIAL RESILIENCE

Human beings are wired for connection. Relationships aren't just emotionally fulfilling—they're biologically essential. Positive social interactions release oxytocin, calm the nervous system, and reduce stress hormones like cortisol. Connection soothes the brain and body, acting as a buffer against life's challenges.

This isn't just a modern phenomenon—it's deeply rooted in our evolution. For thousands of years, humans survived by sticking together in groups. Connection meant safety, security, and access to shared resources, while isolation signaled danger. Even today, our brains and bodies are designed to thrive when surrounded by supportive relationships.

The famous Rat Park experiment offers a striking example of how social connection can transform our responses to pain and stress. In this study, rats were given two water options: one laced with morphine and one plain. When isolated in small, empty cages, the rats drank significantly more of the morphine water. But when they were placed in Rat Park—a stimulating environment filled with other rats and enriching activities—they chose the plain water far more often. Even rats that had previously consumed morphine in isolation reduced their intake once they were moved to Rat Park.

What does this mean for humans? Just like the rats, isolation amplifies stress and discomfort, while connection and a supportive environment calm these responses. For those living with chronic pain, fostering relationships can act as a powerful antidote, helping to soothe the brain and body.

But for those living with chronic pain, maintaining connections can feel like an uphill battle. Pain makes it harder to show up for relationships, and over time, this isolation creates a vicious cycle: Pain → Withdrawal → Stress → Amplified Pain.

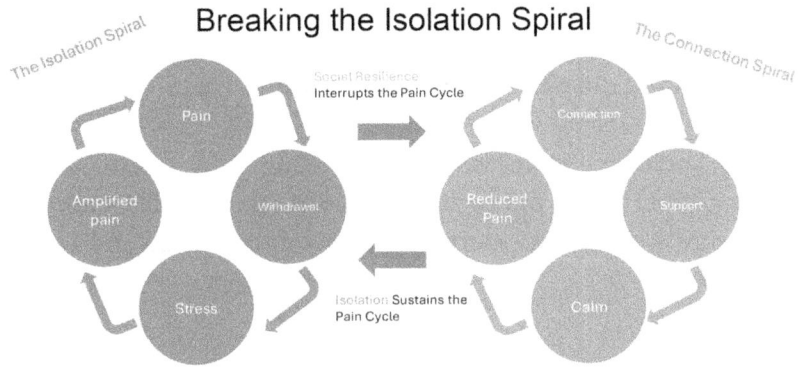

Research even shows that loneliness and isolation activate the same brain regions as physical pain. This means that being socially disconnected doesn't just feel difficult—it amplifies emotional and physical discomfort in measurable ways. On the other hand, fostering connection can calm these neural pathways, reduce the intensity of pain, and create a sense of safety and support that helps you heal.

In this chapter, we'll explore how to build social resilience—a vital pillar of the Peak Resilience Method. You'll discover how meaningful connections don't just reduce isolation but also strengthen your body's ability to heal.

We'll discuss:

- **The Impact of Pain on Relationships**: Understanding how pain can strain your connections and how to navigate these challenges.
- **Rebuilding Trust and Expanding Your Network**: Tools to create a supportive web of relationships, including strategies for repairing old connections and finding new ones.
- **Setting Boundaries for Healthier Relationships**: How to protect your energy by focusing on interactions that uplift you.
- **Daily Practices for Social Resilience**: Small, actionable steps you can take to foster connection and reduce isolation.

Building social resilience isn't about fixing every relationship or becoming more social overnight. It's about taking small, meaningful steps toward a stronger support system that nurtures you and amplifies your healing.

Key Takeaways:
The Power of Connection

Even small moments of connection—like a text or shared meal—can create a ripple effect of resilience.
Building social resilience doesn't mean fixing every relationship; it's about focusing on the ones that matter most.

ADDRESSING COMMON CONCERNS

If the idea of focusing on relationships feels overwhelming, unnecessary, or even weak, you're not alone. You might be thinking:

"I don't want to be a burden." Chronic pain often comes with guilt, but asking for support isn't selfish. In fact, connection is a two-way street—those who care about you often find joy and fulfillment in being there for you.

"Nobody understands what I'm going through." While no one can fully experience your pain, many people can still offer empathy, kindness, and care. Rebuilding connections isn't about perfect understanding—it's about creating bonds that uplift you.

"This feels weak or unimportant." Social resilience isn't "soft." It's a scientifically backed tool that strengthens your nervous system, calms pain pathways, and amplifies your body's ability to heal. Reaching out takes courage, and its benefits are profound.

"I've tried this before, and it didn't work." Connection can take time, and not every relationship can be repaired. But there are new opportunities to explore—whether through support groups, shared activities, or finding new communities.

REBUILDING CONNECTION AFTER SETBACKS

Reconnecting with others after chronic pain has caused withdrawal can feel daunting, but even small steps can create meaningful change. Raj's journey in part four showed us how social resilience isn't about grand gestures—it's about small, intentional actions that rebuild trust and strengthen relationships.

Reaching Out After Silence

For months, Raj had distanced himself from his family. He ignored his sister's texts, convinced she wouldn't understand his pain. But one evening, after reflecting on how isolation had deepened his suffering, he stared at her name on his phone screen. Finally, he typed a simple message:

> *"I know I've been distant. It's not because I don't care. I miss you."*

Her reply came almost instantly:

> *"I miss you too! Let's catch up soon?"*

That short exchange broke through the wall Raj had built. Their first conversation after months of silence wasn't deep or dramatic—they just talked about everyday things. But even that small interaction reminded Raj that he wasn't as alone as he had feared.

Small Gestures, Big Impact

Raj's withdrawal hadn't just affected his family—it had created a quiet tension in his marriage. Meera had always been patient, but Raj knew his silence had left her feeling shut out. One evening, instead of brushing off her concern, he simply said, *"I know I haven't been easy to talk to. Thank you for being here."*

It wasn't an elaborate apology. It wasn't a fix for everything. But Meera's shoulders softened, and she squeezed his hand in response. That small moment reminded Raj that rebuilding connection didn't always require long conversations—sometimes, just acknowledging someone's presence and patience was enough.

He made an effort to show appreciation in small ways. A simple

"Thanks for listening" after she asked about his day. Sitting beside her on the couch instead of retreating to another room. These tiny shifts helped bridge the emotional gap that pain had created.

Finding Community in Unexpected Places

Remember that Raj also found a chronic pain support group online.

At first, he just read other people's posts. Their words felt eerily familiar—the frustration, the isolation, the exhaustion of trying to explain pain to those who couldn't feel it. After weeks of hesitation, Raj finally posted:

"I feel like I've disappeared. I used to be surrounded by people, and now it feels like I don't exist. I don't even know how to explain this to them. Does anyone else feel this way?"

The responses came quickly. Some shared their own stories. Others simply wrote:

"You're not alone."

For the first time in a long time, Raj felt seen. Encouraged by the support, he started engaging more, and eventually, he formed real friendships—connections built on mutual understanding, without the pressure to pretend he was okay.

If pain has strained your relationships, remember: you don't have to solve everything all at once. A single text, a quiet moment of gratitude, or reaching out to someone who understands can be the first step toward rebuilding connection and resilience.

Social resilience is your ability to build and sustain supportive connections, even in the face of challenges like chronic pain. It's about creating a web of relationships—whether with family, friends, or new communities—that strengthens your resilience and supports your healing.

Social resilience isn't just about feeling less alone—it's a cornerstone of your ability to heal and thrive. These connections help reduce stress, calm your nervous system, and create a foundation for lasting resilience.

THE IMPACT OF CHRONIC PAIN ON RELATIONSHIPS

Chronic pain doesn't just affect your body—it can profoundly reshape your relationships. Pain has a way of amplifying misunderstandings, creating emotional distance, and straining even the closest connections. Over time, frustration, guilt, and isolation can take root, leaving you feeling disconnected from the people who matter most.

But it's important to understand that these challenges are not your fault. Pain creates a unique set of obstacles, both for you and for those who care about you. Recognizing how chronic pain affects relationships is the first step toward rebuilding them into sources of strength and support.

KEY CHALLENGES CHRONIC PAIN BRINGS TO RELATIONSHIPS

Emotional and Communication Gaps

Chronic pain often creates an invisible barrier between you and the people in your life. It can be incredibly hard to put the experience of pain into words, especially when it's invisible to others. You may find yourself retreating inward, feeling frustrated or even resentful that your pain is so hard to explain. On the other side, loved ones may struggle to know how to help, sometimes saying the wrong thing or staying silent out of fear of making things worse. This emotional gap can leave both sides feeling misunderstood or disconnected, even when the intention to connect is there.

Shifting Roles and Responsibilities

Pain doesn't just change how you feel—it can change how you show up in your relationships. Tasks you once handled effortlessly might now require help, shifting the balance of responsibilities in your home or family dynamic. You might find yourself leaning more heavily on your partner, friends, or loved ones, which can stir feelings of guilt or worry about being a burden. Meanwhile, those supporting you may feel overwhelmed, unsure of how to strike the balance between helping and maintaining their own energy. These shifting roles can strain even the strongest relationships, but they don't have to define them.

The Pull of Social Withdrawal

Chronic pain often brings an urge to retreat. The thought of attending social events or maintaining plans may feel daunting, especially on days when the pain flares. Over time, the missed dinners and canceled coffee dates can create a widening gulf between you and the people you care about. Friends and loved ones might misinterpret your absence as a lack of interest, leading to fewer invitations and a growing sense of isolation. What begins as a way to conserve energy can inadvertently lead to loneliness, compounding the emotional weight of living with pain.

The Emotional Toll on Loved Ones

Pain doesn't just ripple through your life—it affects those around you in ways that can be both subtle and profound. Partners, children, or close friends might feel helpless in the face of your pain, wanting desperately to fix it but not knowing how. This helplessness can lead to frustration or guilt, sometimes boiling over into arguments or emotional distance. The people who care about you may feel like they're failing, even when they're doing their best to support you. At the same time, you might feel isolated, believing your pain has become a burden on those you love most.

A Path Toward Connection

These challenges are real, and they can feel insurmountable at times. But it's important to remember that while chronic pain may strain relationships, it doesn't have to break them. Acknowledging the ways pain affects your connections is the first step toward rebuilding them. In the next section, we'll explore tools and strategies to strengthen trust, improve communication, and restore the bonds that can help you heal.

THE ROLE OF OXYTOCIN IN SOCIAL RESILIENCE

The Science of Oxytocin: The Bonding Hormone

Oxytocin is a biological superstar when it comes to connection. Often referred to as the "bonding hormone," it plays a central role in fostering trust, emotional safety, and social bonding. But its effects are more than emotional—they're deeply physiological.

When oxytocin is released in your brain, it does several remarkable things:

- **Lowers cortisol levels**, reducing stress and calming the nervous system.
- **Activates the parasympathetic nervous system**, moving your body out of the stress-inducing "fight or flight" state and into "rest and repair."
- **Reinforces feelings of trust and connection**, helping to strengthen relationships and create a sense of safety.

Research shows that oxytocin release from positive social interactions can lower cortisol levels and activate the parasympathetic nervous system, creating a state of relaxation and repair. Studies suggest this hormone may also enhance pain tolerance, making social connection a vital tool in managing chronic pain. This means that oxytocin doesn't just feel good—it helps repair the body and mind from the physiological toll of stress and pain.

Practical Ways to Boost Oxytocin

While oxytocin is often associated with childbirth or romantic bonding, you don't need a special occasion to reap its benefits. Simple, everyday actions can stimulate oxytocin release:

- **Physical Touch**: Hugs, holding hands, or even gentle pats on the back release oxytocin. If touch feels overwhelming, start with something small, like placing your hand on your own chest as a gesture of self-compassion.
- **Shared Laughter**: Humor is a natural oxytocin booster. Watch a comedy special with friends, share a funny memory, or simply let yourself laugh at life's little quirks.
- **Kindness and Gratitude**: Acts of kindness, like helping a neighbor or thanking a loved one, trigger oxytocin. The receiver experiences a boost, too, creating a ripple effect of connection.

"What's one small way you could intentionally create a moment of connection today? Whether it's sharing a laugh, offering a hug, or sending a kind note, every small act strengthens your resilience."

Pharmacological Approaches to Oxytocin

While lifestyle strategies are the most natural and accessible way to foster oxytocin release, there's growing research into pharmacological interventions that may enhance oxytocin's effects.

One promising approach is intranasal oxytocin, delivered via a nasal spray. Studies suggest it may help improve social bonding, reduce stress, and enhance emotional resilience in specific contexts. However, it's important to note that these interventions are still being explored in clinical settings and may not be widely available or appropriate for everyone.

If you're curious about whether pharmacological options could complement your journey, consult with your healthcare provider to discuss their potential role in your treatment plan.

While prescription strategies like intranasal oxytocin are being studied, the foundation of fostering connection remains rooted in everyday actions—touch, laughter, kindness, and shared moments. These small steps create ripples that support both your biology and your relationships.

Oxytocin is more than a hormone—it's a bridge between your biology and your relationships. By fostering it, you're not just creating bonds with others—you're also supporting your body's ability to calm stress and heal from pain. As we explore ways to strengthen trust, rebuild relationships, and expand your social network in the next sections, oxytocin will continue to play a key role in creating the support system you need to thrive.

REBUILDING TRUST AND CONNECTION

Rebuilding relationships after the strain of chronic pain is a journey, not an overnight fix. Whether it's reconnecting with a spouse, opening up to a close friend, or strengthening bonds with family, trust is at the heart of these efforts. Chronic pain might have reshaped some dynamics, but with patience, honesty, and small, consistent actions, you can create a foundation for relationships that uplift and support you.

Start with Open Communication

Connection begins with understanding, and understanding starts with communication. Chronic pain can make it hard to share your feelings, especially if you're used to bottling them up or avoiding conflict. But opening up—even in small ways—can be transformative.

When you're ready to share, start by explaining your experience in simple terms:

- **Describe your pain**: Share what it feels like, how it affects you, and the challenges it creates in your day-to-day life.
- **Express your needs**: Be clear about what kind of support would help, whether it's practical assistance, emotional encouragement, or just listening.
- **Invite collaboration**: Ask for their thoughts or feedback, making it a two-way conversation rather than a monologue.

For example, you might say: "I know my pain sometimes makes me withdraw, and I'm sorry if it's made you feel distant. I'm trying to find better ways to communicate, and I'd love to hear how you've been feeling, too."

"What's one thing you'd like to share with a loved one about your experience with pain? How could you express it in a way that feels true and kind?"

Focus on Small, Consistent Actions

Rebuilding trust doesn't require grand gestures—it's the little things that make the biggest difference. Small, thoughtful actions over time can show your loved ones that you value them and are invested in the relationship.

Here are a few ideas:

- Send a short text to check in or express gratitude.
- Share a moment of humor or positivity, like a funny meme or a story from your day.
- Ask them about their life—taking an interest in their world reminds them that your pain hasn't overshadowed your care for them.

Consistency matters more than perfection. Even if you don't feel up to connecting every day, make an effort when you can, and let your loved ones know that their presence is meaningful to you.

"What's one small action you could take today to show a loved one you care?"

Revisit Old Traditions or Create New Ones

Traditions—whether they're small rituals or big celebrations—give relationships structure and meaning. Chronic pain might have disrupted some of your old traditions, but it's never too late to revisit them or create new ones that work for your current reality.

For example:

- If family game nights became too overwhelming, start with a short card game instead of a long board game.
- If weekend hikes with friends aren't possible, suggest a shorter walk or a relaxing picnic instead.
- Create new traditions like sharing a gratitude moment during dinner or sending weekly check-in texts.

Traditions don't have to be elaborate—they just need to create moments of connection and continuity.

"What's one tradition you'd like to revisit or create with someone you care about?"

Be Honest About Boundaries and Limitations

Honesty is a key ingredient in rebuilding trust, especially when it comes to setting boundaries. Chronic pain often comes with limitations and pretending they don't exist can lead to frustration—for both you and your loved ones.

Being upfront about your boundaries helps create a relationship dynamic that feels safe and sustainable. For example:

- "I'd love to meet up for coffee, but I might need to leave early if my pain flares."
- "I really appreciate you offering to help, but I'd prefer to handle this on my own today."

Setting boundaries isn't about pushing people away—it's about ensuring that your relationships are built on mutual respect and understanding.

"What's one boundary you'd like to communicate in a relationship, and how could you share it in a caring way?"

Rebuilding Together

Rebuilding relationships is a collaborative effort. By practicing open communication, taking small actions, and honoring traditions and boundaries, you can create a foundation of trust and mutual support. Relationships strained by chronic pain aren't broken—they're evolving. With patience and intention, they can grow into something stronger and more resilient than before.

Finding New Sources of Support

While rebuilding existing relationships is important, chronic pain often creates opportunities—or even a need—to find new sources of connection. Support doesn't have to come solely from the people already in your life. Expanding your social network can introduce fresh perspectives, shared experiences, and connections that are uniquely suited to this stage of your journey.

Building new relationships may feel daunting, especially if pain has limited your energy or mobility, but even small steps can create ripples of change.

Expanding your social connections helps fill the gaps left by strained or distant relationships. It also introduces you to people who understand your experiences on a deeper level or share similar challenges. Joining communities—whether virtual or in-person—can:

- **Boost oxytocin and reduce stress** by fostering trust and connection.
- **Provide a sense of belonging**, which counteracts the isolating effects of pain.
- **Offer emotional and practical support**, such as coping strategies or resources for managing chronic pain.

Exploring Online Communities

The rise of online communities has created powerful spaces where people with shared experiences can connect, learn, and support each other. These platforms allow you to:

- **Share Your Story**: Expressing your thoughts and challenges in a supportive space can be cathartic and help others feel less alone.
- **Learn New Strategies**: Members often share tools, techniques, and insights that might be helpful in managing your own journey.
- **Connect Without Pressure**: Online interactions can be paced according to your energy and comfort, making them accessible even on difficult days.

Pro Tip

When exploring online communities, look for spaces with clear guidelines for respectful engagement and active moderation. Communities with supportive, solution-focused discussions tend to foster the best connections. Avoid spaces dominated by negativity or unproductive venting, as these can reinforce feelings of isolation or frustration.

Other Opportunities to Build Connection

In addition to online communities, you might consider exploring these options:

- **Shared Interest Communities**: Whether it's art, gardening, or photography, engaging in hobbies can connect you with like-minded individuals while giving you a creative outlet.
- **Volunteering Opportunities**: Helping others can reduce stress and provide a sense of purpose. Even small contributions to causes you care about can create meaningful interactions.

How to Start Small

Finding new sources of support doesn't have to mean diving headfirst into a large group or committing to regular meetups. Here are some small steps to get started:

- **Join an Online Forum or Group**: Introduce yourself by sharing your story or participating in discussions that resonate with you.
- **Attend One Virtual Event**: Look for an online workshop, webinar, or support meeting that aligns with your interests or needs.
- **Combine Connection with Low-Energy Activities**: Try participating in activities that match your current

energy level, like joining a casual book club or crafting group.

Pro Tip

Start with what feels manageable and safe. The goal is to create opportunities for connection, not overwhelm yourself.

"What's one new group, activity, or online community you'd like to explore? How could this help you feel more connected?"

Reframing the Idea of Support

Support doesn't have to look the same for everyone. For some, it may mean deep conversations in an online community. For others, it could involve shared laughter in a hobby class or the quiet solidarity of a virtual group. Whatever form it takes, the key is creating a web of connection that uplifts and sustains you.

Setting Boundaries for Healthy Relationships

Healthy relationships are built on mutual respect and understanding, but chronic pain can sometimes blur the lines between support and strain. Setting boundaries is essential—not just to protect your energy, but also to ensure that your relationships remain sources of strength rather than stress.

Boundaries aren't about pushing people away. Instead, they're about creating a framework where both you and your loved ones can thrive. They allow you to be honest about your limitations while maintaining connection and trust.

Why Boundaries Matter

Boundaries are especially important for people living with chronic pain because:

- Energy Is Limited: Pain already takes a toll on your physical and emotional resources, so conserving energy is crucial.
- Healthy Relationships Require Balance: Overextending yourself—or allowing others to overstep—can lead to frustration, resentment, or burnout.
- Boundaries Promote Understanding: Being clear about your needs helps loved ones support you in ways that are truly helpful, reducing misunderstandings and stress.

How to Set Boundaries with Compassion

Boundaries are most effective when they're communicated clearly and kindly. Here's a framework to help you navigate these conversations:

1. Acknowledge the Relationship: Start by affirming the importance of your connection. For example:
   - "I really value the time we spend together."
   - "Your support means so much to me."
2. State Your Needs Honestly: Be direct but gentle about what you need. Avoid overexplaining or apologizing. For example:
   - "I'd love to meet up, but I may need to leave early if my pain flares."
   - "I appreciate your help, but I need some time to rest before we talk again."
3. Reassure Them: Let the other person know that your boundary isn't a rejection. For example:
   - "This doesn't mean I don't enjoy spending time with you—it just helps me take care of myself."

Pro Tip

Practice these conversations when you're feeling calm, so you're prepared if emotions run high later.

Look back at Raj, for example. When his pain flared, he often agreed to social plans he didn't have the energy for, fearing he'd let people down. Over time, this left him feeling drained and resentful, and his relationships grew strained. After learning to set boundaries, he tried saying, "I'd love to meet up, but I may need to leave early if I'm not feeling up to it." At first, he worried friends would feel rejected, but to his surprise, they were understanding. Setting clear limits allowed Raj to show up authentically, and his relationships became stronger as a result.

Common Boundary Scenarios and How to Handle Them

When You Need to Say No

It's okay to decline requests or invitations that feel overwhelming. Try saying:

- "I really appreciate the invitation, but I need to rest today. Can we reschedule?"
- "I'd love to help, but I'm not able to take this on right now."

When Loved Ones Don't Understand Your Pain

If someone questions or dismisses your experience, respond calmly and assertively:

- "I know it's hard to understand what I'm going through, but I hope you can trust that I'm doing my best to manage."
- "Pain is unpredictable, and it's hard for me to explain exactly how it feels. Thank you for being patient with me."

When Relationships Feel Draining

It's important to recognize when certain relationships consistently leave you feeling worse. Setting firm boundaries might sound like this:

- "I value our relationship, but I need to step back from conversations that feel overwhelming for me right now."
- "I need to focus on my well-being, so I'm taking some space to recharge."

"What's one boundary you need to set in a relationship, and how can you express it with honesty and compassion?"

Boundaries as Acts of Strength

Setting boundaries isn't about limiting your relationships—it's about strengthening them. By being honest about your needs and respecting your own limits, you create the conditions for healthier, more balanced connections. When relationships are built on mutual understanding and respect, they become powerful sources of resilience that support you on your healing journey.

Setting boundaries isn't just about managing energy or preserving relationships—it's about creating the emotional space to rediscover what truly matters to you. Boundaries free up your mental and physical capacity to focus on the people, goals, and activities that align with your mission. In the next section, we'll explore how to reconnect with that mission and align your relationships to support it.

SOCIAL RESILIENCE AND YOUR MISSION

Chronic pain has a way of narrowing your world, making it feel as though your life revolves around managing discomfort and limitations. Social resilience, however, can help you look beyond pain and reconnect with what matters most: your mission. Your mission is your "why"—the driving force that gives your life meaning and purpose.

Strong relationships play a crucial role in supporting this journey. They remind you that you're more than your pain, helping you re-engage with your passions, goals, and the unique contributions only you can make.

How Social Resilience Connects to Your Mission

Social connections don't just buffer stress—they can also reignite your sense of purpose. Here's how:

- **Encouragement to Dream Bigger**: Supportive relationships can inspire you to think beyond your immediate challenges and focus on long-term goals.
- **Accountability and Motivation**: Sharing your goals with trusted people creates a sense of accountability, making it easier to stay on track.
- **A Safety Net for Risk-Taking**: Knowing you have a strong support system gives you the confidence to pursue meaningful challenges, even if they involve setbacks or uncertainty.

For example, someone in a supportive circle of friends may feel empowered to start a small side business, volunteer for a cause they care about, or take steps toward a long-held creative dream.

Zooming Out to Reframe Your Mission

When pain limits what you once thought was your purpose, it can feel like you've lost a piece of yourself. But your mission isn't tied to a single activity—it's about the core values and meaning behind that activity. By zooming out and looking at the bigger picture, you can often find new ways to fulfill your purpose, even if the methods look different than before.

For example:

- If you believed your mission was to create art but chronic pain makes it difficult to draw, you might reframe your purpose as sharing art with others. This could mean mentoring young artists, organizing community art projects, or teaching others to appreciate the power of creativity.
- If you thought your mission was to run marathons, but pain limits your ability to train, your purpose might really be about inspiring perseverance and wellness. You could achieve this by supporting others' fitness journeys, coaching beginners, or fundraising for health-related causes.

Reframing doesn't mean giving up on what matters—it means broadening your perspective to find new ways of living your values.

Just as reframing your mission allows you to rediscover purpose and alignment, rebuilding social connections creates the supportive framework needed to pursue it. Relationships, whether old or new, act as anchors that hold you steady as you take steps toward a fulfilling and resilient life.

Sharing Your Mission with Others

Once you've clarified your mission, share it with trusted people who can support and encourage you. Talking about your dreams, even in small ways, strengthens your commitment to them and invites others to become part of your journey.

For example, you might say:

- "I've been thinking about how much I miss painting, and I'd like to set up a small studio at home. Would you be willing to help me get started?"
- "I've always wanted to volunteer for [a cause], and I'm

trying to figure out how to make it work with my energy levels. I'd love your advice."

By sharing your mission, you allow others to offer encouragement and collaboration, turning your goals into a shared effort.

Building Collaborative Traditions

Relationships thrive on shared experiences. By creating new traditions that align with your mission, you strengthen both your sense of purpose and your connections with others.

Examples include:

- Planning monthly check-ins with a friend to discuss progress on your personal goals.
- Inviting loved ones to join you in activities that reflect your passions, like volunteering, exercising, or learning something new together.
- Starting small rituals, like sharing a gratitude practice or dedicating a specific day each month to a meaningful activity.

These shared traditions provide structure and continuity, reinforcing your mission as a central part of your life.

How to Zoom Out and Reframe

Here's a process to help you identify your mission's deeper meaning:

1. **Identify the Core Value:** What is the underlying value or emotion that your passion brings you? For example:
   - Drawing cartoons might represent creativity, joy, or connection.
   - Running marathons might symbolize discipline, achievement, or inspiration.

2. **Look for New Expressions:** Once you've identified the core value, think about how else you could express it in your life. Ask yourself:
   - "What other activities align with this value?"
   - "How could I share this value with others in a meaningful way?"
3. **Take Small Steps:** Test out different ways to live your mission. For example, if your mission shifts from drawing cartoons to teaching art, you could start by volunteering at a local school or mentoring a single student.

"What is the deeper meaning behind your passion or goal? How could you adapt this purpose in a way that aligns with your current abilities?"

Your mission isn't tied to a single skill or achievement—it's about the values and impact that define who you are. Chronic pain might change how you express your mission, but it doesn't erase your purpose. By zooming out, sharing your goals with others, and building traditions that reflect your values, you can bring your mission to life in ways you never imagined.

MAKING SOCIAL RESILIENCE A DAILY PRACTICE

Social resilience isn't built overnight—it's cultivated through small, consistent actions over time. Just as you would exercise your body or practice mindfulness to strengthen other aspects of resilience, nurturing your relationships requires regular effort. These daily practices aren't about perfection; they're about creating habits that support meaningful connection, reduce isolation, and reinforce your ability to heal.

Strong relationships act like a safety net, cushioning you against stress and amplifying your resilience. But relationships, like muscles, need regular care to grow and thrive. Daily practices:

- **Reinforce Connection:** Small gestures keep relationships alive, even when time or energy is limited.
- **Reduce Stress:** Regular interaction with supportive people calms the nervous system, lowers cortisol levels, and fosters a sense of security.
- **Strengthen Longevity:** Consistent effort builds trust and ensures relationships remain strong, even during tough times.

Simple, Impactful Daily Practices

Making social resilience part of your routine doesn't have to be complicated. Here are practical ideas to weave connection into your daily life:

Start the Day with Gratitude

Each morning, reflect on someone in your life you're grateful for and why. This sets a positive tone for the day and fosters appreciation for your relationships.

- **Send a Gratitude Text**: Send a quick message to the person you're grateful for, letting them know you're thinking of them.

Reach Out to One Person Each Day

Connection doesn't require long conversations. A short text, a quick phone call, or a comment on social media can remind someone you care.

- **Reach out and Connect**: Set a goal to connect with one person daily, even if it's just to check in or say hello.

Combine Connection with Restorative Activities

Social resilience can overlap with activities that restore you physically or emotionally. For example, invite a friend to join you for a gentle walk, a yoga class, or a shared meal.

- **Combine Connection with Activity**: Schedule one shared activity per week that brings joy to you and someone you care about.

Reflect on Your Progress

Take time at the end of the week to reflect on your connections. Jot down one moment of connection. What felt meaningful? What could you do differently next week? Reflection deepens your awareness of the positive impact of social resilience.

Helpful Tools

Consider using a journal, habit tracker, or app to record your social connections and meaningful moments. Apps like Daylio or MoodNotes can track emotions and highlight patterns, while a simple calendar can remind you to reach out to someone each day. These tools can make your progress tangible and help you stay consistent.

__Journaling Prompts__: "Which relationships in your life bring you joy? How can you nurture those connections?"

"What's one small action you can take today to reconnect with someone meaningful?"

"What's one small action you could take today to nurture a connection in your life? How could this become part of your daily or weekly routine?"

A RIPPLE EFFECT OF RESILIENCE

Small, consistent actions in your social life can create profound ripple effects, strengthening your relationships and deepening your resilience. By making connection a daily practice, you're not only nurturing your relationships—you're reinforcing the foundation for healing, growth, and thriving.

Social resilience isn't just a nice idea—it's a powerful tool that strengthens your ability to heal and thrive. By fostering connection, setting boundaries, and finding new sources of support, you're creating a foundation for relationships that uplift and empower you. These connections remind you that you're not alone, offering strength, encouragement, and inspiration as you move forward.

But social resilience is more than emotional support—it's a biological force that helps rewire your internal systems. Positive social interactions calm the nervous system, lower stress hormones, and even reduce pain perception. Studies suggest that social bonding helps shift the body out of "fight or flight" mode, reducing activity in the amygdala (the brain's fear center) and increasing activation in areas linked to trust and safety. Over time, these changes can help reverse the chronic stress responses that amplify pain. Every meaningful connection you build is a step toward reversing the chronic pain state and bringing your body back into balance.

By fostering connection, you're not just strengthening your relationships—you're also healing the disrupted internal systems that chronic pain affects. Each moment of trust, support, and shared laughter helps calm your nervous system, reduce stress responses, and create the conditions for repair and growth.

Affirmation: *Every connection I nurture strengthens my resilience. I am not alone in this journey.*

Small, consistent efforts—like reaching out to someone you trust, reflecting on your mission, or sharing a simple moment of gratitude—

can spark profound ripples in your life. Social resilience is about more than reducing isolation; it's about building a life filled with purpose, belonging, and mutual care.

As an example, consider Raj. Like many of our patients, he'd spent years feeling isolated, convinced that no one truly understood what he was going through. But with small, consistent efforts—joining an online support group, sending a simple *"I miss you"* text to his sister, and making a habit of acknowledging Meera's quiet support—he slowly began to rebuild his connections. One day, he realized that while his pain was still there, it no longer defined him. His relationships, his sense of purpose, and the connections he had nurtured became the anchors that grounded him, reminding him that resilience wasn't just about enduring pain—it was about finding ways to live fully despite it.,

With social resilience firmly in place, it's time to consider one final element to help you bring together everything you've learned into a personalized plan: the power of mindset.

CHAPTER 16
THE MINDSET SHIFT: UNLOCKING RESILIENCE THROUGH THE POWER OF BELIEF

Your mindset—the beliefs and attitudes you hold about yourself and your challenges—has a profound effect on your health. This isn't just motivational talk; it's grounded in science. Research led by Dr. Alia Crum at Stanford University shows that mindsets actively shape how your body responds to the world around you. They influence everything from stress levels to immune function, and yes, even how you experience pain.

What sets mindset science apart is its ability to connect our thoughts to real physiological outcomes. Consider the placebo effect: countless studies have shown that people who believe they are receiving an effective treatment often experience real, measurable improvements—even when the treatment is inert. This isn't a trick of the mind; it's a demonstration of the brain's ability to influence healing.

Dr. Crum's work expands on this concept with stress mindset theory. Her research shows that people who view stress as a challenge rather than a threat experience lower cortisol levels, less inflammation, and improved resilience. This shift in mindset fundamentally changes how the body reacts to stress, and similar principles can be applied to pain.

We already know that pain isn't simply a physical sensation; it's also shaped by how your brain interprets signals from your body. When you see pain as a threat, it amplifies stress and tension, locking you into a cycle of suffering. But what if you could reframe your mindset about pain? Shifting your perspective from "pain-as-threat" to "pain-as-signal" has the power to transform how your brain processes discomfort.

You may remember from earlier chapters how neuroplasticity helps reshape thought patterns and emotional responses. In this chapter, we take that concept further by exploring how your mindset influences specific brain regions involved in pain perception. This includes activating areas like the prefrontal cortex, which dampens pain signals, and quieting areas like the amygdala, which amplifies them.

Reflection Prompt: *Think about a belief you hold about your pain. How might you reframe it into something more supportive? For example, "This pain is ruining my day" could become "This pain is a signal to rest and care for my body."*

This isn't just a mental exercise; it creates tangible, physical changes in your brain that help break the cycle of chronic pain.

Mindset influences more than your brain; it also affects your body's stress and inflammatory responses. Negative beliefs about pain increase stress hormones like cortisol, heightening sensitivity to pain and slowing recovery. By shifting those beliefs, you lower cortisol levels, reduce inflammation, and create a healing environment within your body.

This isn't about dismissing pain or pretending it doesn't exist. Pain is real, but so is your capacity to change how you relate to it. By embracing a mindset that views pain as a guide—a messenger asking for attention and care—you can take the first step toward reclaiming control.

What's one belief you hold about your pain that might be influencing how you experience it? How could you reframe that belief to support healing?

> **Key Takeaways:**
> **How Mindset Affects Pain**
> Beliefs about pain shape how the brain processes discomfort. Viewing pain as a signal for growth reduces stress and fosters resilience. Reframing stress as a challenge (rather than a threat) lowers cortisol and inflammation.
> Small mindset shifts, practiced consistently, can create long-lasting changes in how pain is experienced.

PRACTICAL STRATEGIES FOR REFRAMING PAIN

Pain is often seen as the enemy—something to avoid, suppress, or fight against. But what if pain could be something else entirely? Instead of viewing it as a limitation, you could see it as a signal, a teacher, or even a catalyst for growth. Shifting your mindset in this way doesn't deny the reality of pain—it transforms how you interact with it.

In this section, we'll explore practical strategies to help you reframe your relationship with pain, using proven techniques like journaling, visualization, and stress reappraisal. These approaches are designed to give you tools to turn pain into a guide, rather than an obstacle.

Pain is your body's way of communicating that something needs attention. Instead of viewing it as purely a threat, what if you could see it as a signal asking for change? This doesn't mean the pain is easy or welcome, but it does mean it can be informative.

Consider Lisa from part two. By journaling about their pain, Lisa began noticing patterns—moments of tension during meetings or after long hours at the computer. This awareness helped her make small but impactful adjustments, like standing up to stretch every hour or scheduling shorter, more focused work sessions. By reframing their pain as a signal, Lisa moved from feeling helpless to taking constructive action.

If journaling feels unfamiliar or difficult at first, start small. Even writing one sentence about what your pain might be asking for can provide valuable insights. There's no right or wrong way to reflect—what matters is beginning the practice.

Try This

At the end of each day, take five minutes to journal about your pain. Ask yourself:

- What was I doing or feeling when I noticed the pain?
- What might my body be trying to tell me?
- What small change could I make to respond to this signal?

From Limitation to Transformation

Pain often feels like a wall—something that blocks you from living the life you want. But what if that wall could become a stepping stone? Athletes often lean into discomfort as a way to grow stronger, reframing their effort as an investment in their goals. You can do the same with chronic pain.

Earlier in the book, we introduced mindfulness and gratitude as tools for cultivating emotional balance. Here, we'll explore how these practices, when paired with a growth-oriented mindset, can transform your relationship with pain. Visualization, for example, isn't just about imagining relief—it's about using your mindset to shift how your brain processes discomfort, reinforcing resilience through intentional focus.

One powerful way to shift your perspective is through visualization. Imagine your pain as an obstacle on a hiking trail. At first, it may seem insurmountable. But with each step, you learn to navigate the terrain, finding new strength and clarity as you climb. By visualizing yourself overcoming these challenges, you can shift your mindset from one of defeat to one of empowerment.

Try This

Find a quiet space and sit comfortably. Close your eyes and imagine yourself navigating a challenge. Picture yourself moving through it with strength and focus, feeling more resilient and capable with each step. When you finish, take a moment to notice how your mindset has shifted.

GROWTH THROUGH DISCOMFORT

Discomfort is a part of life, but it doesn't have to be a dead end. Dr. Alia Crum's work on stress reappraisal shows that viewing stress as a tool for growth changes how the body responds to it—lowering cortisol levels and improving performance. The same principle applies to pain.

Think of times in your life when discomfort led to growth—a tough conversation that deepened a relationship or a challenging project that helped you develop new skills. Pain, like those moments, can push you to adapt in ways you didn't think possible.

Try This

Write a letter to yourself about a time when you overcame discomfort or pain in the past. What did you learn from that experience? How did it shape you? Then, consider how those lessons could apply to the challenges you're facing now.

> *What's one strategy—journaling, visualization, or reappraisal—that resonates most with you? How can you start using it today to reframe your relationship with pain?*

MINDSET AND BIOLOGICAL RESILIENCE

Your body responds to what your mind believes. Dr. Alia Crum's groundbreaking hotel maid study provides a powerful illustration. Maids at a hotel were split into two groups: one group was informed that their daily work—vacuuming, lifting, walking—met the surgeon general's recommendations for exercise, while the other group received no such information. Remarkably, after just four weeks, the maids who believed they were exercising showed measurable improvements in their weight, blood pressure, and body composition, even though their actual activity levels hadn't changed.

The reason beliefs influence physiological outcomes lies in the brain's role as a regulator. When you believe an action—like movement or rest—is beneficial, your brain adjusts hormonal and neural responses to align with that belief. This can mean lowering cortisol, reducing inflammation, or enhancing the release of endorphins. In essence, your brain translates belief into biological signals, amplifying the effects of your actions.

MINDSET AND PSYCHOLOGICAL RESILIENCE

Dr. Crum's research on stress mindset theory further highlights the power of perspective. In one study, participants were shown videos framing stress as either harmful or beneficial. Those who adopted the belief that stress could enhance performance experienced lower cortisol levels, better cardiovascular responses, and improved focus.

This concept translates directly to how you view pain. If you see pain as purely harmful, it reinforces fear and avoidance, creating a cycle of suffering. But if you reframe pain as a signal for adaptation or growth, your brain can begin to modulate those signals differently, dampening their intensity and fostering resilience. This shift in perspective activates the brain's pain modulation networks, including the prefrontal cortex, which helps regulate discomfort and emotional responses.

MINDSET AND SOCIAL RESILIENCE

Mindset can even influence how we connect with others. Studies have shown that when people believe social interactions are opportunities for growth and mutual support, they experience increased feelings of connection and reduced stress. This aligns with research on oxytocin, often called the "bonding hormone," which is released during positive social interactions and helps calm the nervous system.

In Chapter 14, we discussed the importance of social resilience and the role of connection in healing. Mindset enhances this process by influencing how you perceive relationships. Viewing connections as sources of collaboration rather than burden helps you tap into the biological benefits of social support, such as oxytocin release and reduced stress.

Think about an area of your life—biological, psychological, or social—where a shift in mindset could amplify your efforts. What belief could you reframe today to make your actions more impactful?

These principles aren't just theoretical—they're tools that real people have used to transform their lives. Let's explore a few stories of individuals who embraced mindset shifts to overcome chronic pain and regain their sense of purpose.

STORIES OF TRANSFORMATION: THE POWER OF MINDSET SHIFTS

Seeing how others have transformed their lives through mindset shifts can help us realize what's possible in our own journey. The following stories highlight the power of reframing pain, demonstrating how small but consistent changes in perspective can lead to profound results.

A Professional Athlete Reclaims Strength

When Mia, a marathon runner, developed chronic Achilles tendon pain, it felt like her world was ending. Running had always been her outlet, her joy, and her identity. But now, even a short jog left her limping in frustration.

At first, Mia focused on what she couldn't do, replaying the thought: *"If I can't run, who am I?"* Her mindset left her feeling stuck and defeated. But her coach introduced her to the concept of reframing. What if the pain wasn't a punishment but a message from her body, asking for change?

Mia began shifting her perspective. She adjusted her training to include swimming and yoga, learning to appreciate the strength she was building in other areas. Journaling helped her uncover limiting beliefs about needing to "push through" pain, and she replaced them with empowering ones, like *"Rest is part of resilience."* Over time, her Achilles improved, but more importantly, Mia discovered a deeper sense of strength and balance that extended beyond running.

By reframing her beliefs about rest and recovery, Mia's brain likely shifted focus from amplifying pain signals to engaging its pain regulation systems. This mental shift activated neuroplasticity, enabling her to retrain her responses to discomfort and reinforce new, healthier patterns of movement and rest.

An Executive Finds Focus Through Adaptation

Ethan, a high-performing executive in the tech world, spent years ignoring his lower back pain. Long hours at his desk and a relentless travel schedule left him exhausted, but he told himself: *"I just have to push harder."*

When the pain began interfering with his ability to lead meetings and travel, Ethan finally sought help. His physical therapist encouraged him to view his pain as feedback rather than failure. Through guided visualization, Ethan started imagining his back pain as a red flag on his dashboard—a signal that he needed to adjust his routine rather than push harder.

This mindset shift prompted Ethan to experiment with standing meetings, stretch breaks, and more intentional downtime. The results were transformative. Not only did his back pain improve, but Ethan found himself more focused and present at work, setting a tone of resilience for his team.

A Creative Professional Finds a New Path

Sofia, a graphic designer, faced an even greater challenge. After developing debilitating hand pain, her ability to draw and design—the core of her work—was severely limited. For months, she fought against the pain, forcing herself to work long hours until the pain was unbearable.

Eventually, Sofia realized that her current approach wasn't sustainable. A friend suggested she think about her mission more broadly. What if her work wasn't just about *creating art* but about *inspiring creativity in others*?

This shift opened new doors. Sofia began mentoring young artists, helping them develop their skills and find their voice. Though she still faced limitations with her hands, her pain no longer defined her. Instead, it became the turning point that led her to a mission she found even more fulfilling.

Think about a challenge or limitation in your own life. What would it look like to reframe it as an opportunity? What small steps could you take today to start transforming the way you approach it?

INTEGRATING MINDSET SCIENCE INTO THE RESILIENCE CODE

Mindset isn't just one piece of the puzzle—it's the thread that weaves through every aspect of your resilience journey. As you've learned throughout this book, the Resilience Code is built on the three pillars of biological, psychological, and social resilience. Your mindset influences how you engage with each of these areas, amplifying the effectiveness of the tools and strategies you've already explored.

Mindset and Biological Resilience

Your body responds to what your mind believes. When you view your efforts—like restorative movement, improved sleep hygiene, or anti-inflammatory nutrition—as steps toward healing rather than chores or obligations, your mindset primes your body to benefit more fully. Research shows that positive beliefs about health behaviors, such as exercise or healthy eating, enhance their physiological effects.

For example, if you see exercise as painful or burdensome, your stress response might kick in, increasing cortisol levels and reducing the activity of pain-modulating systems. But when you shift your perspective to view movement as a form of healing or empowerment, your body responds differently, releasing endorphins and calming the nervous system.

Mindset and Psychological Resilience

The psychological tools you've explored—like mindfulness, gratitude, and reframing—are most effective when paired with a growth-oriented mindset. For example, mindfulness isn't just a practice; it's an opportunity to explore the stories you tell yourself about pain. Are those stories helping you heal, or are they keeping you stuck?

By approaching these tools with curiosity and self-compassion, you strengthen the neural pathways that support positive thinking and emotional regulation. This reinforces the changes you're working toward and helps you build momentum, even on tough days.

Mindset and Social Resilience

Our beliefs about relationships can shape how we connect with others. If you view yourself as a burden because of your pain, you may withdraw, creating a barrier to the support you need. But if you reframe your perspective—seeing relationships as mutual and collaborative—you open the door to deeper connection.

Mindset shifts can also enhance how you approach social supports. For instance, instead of seeing a support group as a last resort, you could view it as a space to share strength and insights. This reframing fosters connection and helps you tap into the healing power of community.

Bringing It All Together

As you build your Resilience Code, mindset acts as the foundation that supports every strategy and action. It's what transforms your efforts into meaningful, lasting change. By aligning your beliefs with your goals, you create a pathway to thrive—not just beyond pain, but in every area of your life.

Take a moment to reflect on the pillars of your Resilience Code—biological, psychological, and social. What role does mindset currently play in each area? What's one belief you could shift to amplify your efforts?

YOUR MINDSET SHIFT CHECKLIST

Your mindset is more than just a set of beliefs—it's the foundation for building resilience across every area of your life. By shifting how you think about pain, you can unlock the power to heal, adapt, and thrive. This chapter has shown you how to reframe pain, view it as a signal for growth, and integrate mindset science into your Resilience Code. Now it's time to put these concepts into action.

Here are a few steps to help you begin transforming your mindset today:

1. **Challenge Negative Beliefs**

If you often think, *"This pain will never get better,"* pause and ask yourself: *"Is this belief entirely true? What evidence suggests it might not be?"* You might realize that while the pain has been persistent, there have been moments of improvement or tools that have provided relief.

2. **Practice Reframing Pain as a Signal**

Imagine that your pain is asking for your attention—not to punish you, but to guide you. For instance, shoulder tension might be a sign to take breaks from your desk or to stretch more often. By viewing pain as feedback, you can identify changes that help your body recover.

3. **Visualize Growth Through Discomfort**

Spend 5–10 minutes imagining yourself overcoming challenges. Picture your resilience building with every step forward.

4. **Track Your Mindset Shifts**

Keep a log of moments when you successfully reframed pain or approached a situation with a growth-oriented mindset. Reflect on how these changes influenced your day.

5. **Engage in Daily Mindset Practices**

Integrate mindfulness, gratitude, or affirmations into your routine to strengthen your ability to focus on the positive and stay grounded during difficult moments.

Try These Today

- **Morning Affirmation**: Start your day with a statement like, "I have the strength to navigate today's challenges."
- **Midday Check-In**: Pause for a moment to ask yourself: "What is my pain trying to tell me? How can I respond with care?"
- **Evening Gratitude**: Reflect on one thing that brought you comfort or joy during the day, no matter how small.

Mindset work isn't about pretending pain doesn't exist—it's about taking control of how you respond to it. Each time you reframe a negative belief, view pain as a guide, or choose growth over fear, you're strengthening your resilience. This journey requires courage and consistency, but the rewards are profound.

Imagine a future where pain no longer defines you—where your actions, choices, and relationships reflect your strength and adaptability. This isn't just possible; it's achievable when you take the first step toward shifting your mindset.

Think back to Sarah from our introduction. Or to Emma and Maria from part one, Lisa from part two, Andre from part three, and Raj from part four. All of their journeys began with frustration and defeat. By shifting their mindset and viewing pain as a signal for growth, they found clarity and balance—not by erasing the pain, but by learning to respond to it differently. Like them, you have the power to take these small, intentional steps and create a life that feels purposeful and resilient.

Affirmation: *I have the power to reshape my response to pain. Each small shift in my mindset brings me closer to resilience and healing.*

Throughout this book, we've explored the interconnected pillars of resilience—biological, psychological, and social. We've tied those threads together, showing how mindset amplifies your efforts in each area. With mindset as your foundation, you'll be ready to align your biological, psychological, and social strategies into a plan that supports your growth and recovery.

In our final chapter, we'll build on this foundation by helping you design your personalized Resilience Code—a roadmap for integrating everything you've learned into a framework tailored to your unique journey.

CHAPTER 17
YOUR RESILIENCE CODE STARTS NOW

When it comes to chronic pain, resilience isn't a one-size-fits-all solution. Pain affects everyone differently—your triggers, your strengths, and your resources are unique. That's why copying someone else's approach to healing rarely works. What worked for your friend or a story you read online might leave you feeling stuck or frustrated.

Creating a personalized plan—the Resilience Code—isn't about following a checklist. It's a framework, designed to help you reflect on your experiences, understand your challenges, and choose strategies that fit your life. Your Resilience Code becomes your guide, helping you take consistent, meaningful steps toward healing while staying aligned with your values and goals.

Why does personalization matter so much? Consider some of the patients we've met in these pages. Lisa, Andre, and Raj—while all three of the components of their biopsychosocial systems were under attack from chronic pain, for each a different system was the primary culprit. For Lisa, prioritizing biological resilience was the key, where Andre found that psychological resilience was his weak point in the pain chain. As we've established, chronic pain doesn't just disrupt one system—it affects many interconnected parts of your body and life. Your nervous system, immune response, endocrine function, and even your relationships can fall out of sync, creating a vicious cycle that reinforces pain. To truly heal, you need a framework that rebuilds balance across all these areas, one step at a time, and prioritizes the system (or systems) most responsible for flare ups.

That's where personalization comes in.

Biological Resilience: What works for one person—like high-intensity exercise or an anti-inflammatory diet—may need to be adapted or simplified for someone else.

Psychological Resilience: Reframing negative thoughts might feel easy for some but overwhelming for others.

Social Resilience: Not everyone has access to strong support networks, but there are always ways to nurture connection.

The key is starting where you are and focusing on what feels achievable right now. Small, consistent actions tailored to your needs will create lasting change.

In this chapter, you'll learn how to:

- Reflect on your current strengths and challenges using the biopsychosocial framework.
- Set clear, actionable goals that align with your life and values.
- Use tools like the Resilience Wheel to track your progress and adapt your plan over time.

Your Resilience Code isn't just about managing pain—it's about reclaiming your mission and rediscovering what makes you feel alive.

"What's one area of your life where you feel the most stuck right now? What's one small step that could help you move forward?"

ASSESSING YOUR BIOPSYCHOSOCIAL PROFILE

Before creating your Resilience Code, it's essential to understand where you are right now. Assessing your biopsychosocial profile—the interconnected biological, psychological, and social factors that influence your health—helps you identify both your strengths and the areas that might need the most attention.

This process isn't about judgment or perfection. It's about gaining clarity and using that knowledge to take meaningful, achievable steps forward. By reflecting on how chronic pain has affected these three pillars of resilience, you'll create a solid foundation for personal growth and healing.

Biological Resilience

Your biological resilience is tied to how well your body is functioning. Chronic pain can disrupt your nervous system, immune function, and endocrine balance, creating a state of constant stress. Questions to consider:

- "Do I wake up feeling rested and refreshed most days?"
- "How often do I move my body in ways that feel good or manageable?"
- "Do I notice patterns between what I eat or drink and how I feel?"

"What's one small change I could make to support my body's healing process (e.g., better sleep, improved hydration, or gentle movement)?"

Psychological Resilience

Psychological resilience focuses on how well you manage thoughts, emotions, and stress. Chronic pain often rewires the brain, creating patterns of fear, frustration, and negative self-talk. Questions to consider:

- "How often do I find myself stuck in negative thought loops about my pain?"
- "Do I have strategies in place to calm my mind during stressful moments?"
- "Do I feel a sense of purpose or hope, even on challenging days?"

___

"What's one way I could support my mental well-being this week (e.g., practicing mindfulness, journaling, or seeking support)?"

___

Social Resilience

Social resilience reflects the quality and depth of your connections with others. Pain can isolate you, making it harder to maintain relationships or build new ones. Questions to consider:

- "Do I feel supported by my relationships with family or friends?"
- "Are there times when I feel lonely or disconnected, even in a group?"
- "What's one step I could take to build or strengthen a connection?"

___

"What's one relationship in my life that brings me joy or comfort? How can I nurture that connection?"

___

Visualize Your Resilience

Use the Resilience Wheel to map out your strengths and areas for growth. Divide the wheel into three sections—Biological, Psychological, and Social—and shade in each section based on how strong you feel in that area (e.g., a score of 7/10 means shading in 70% of that section). This visual snapshot will help you identify which pillar needs the most focus as you start building your Resilience Code.

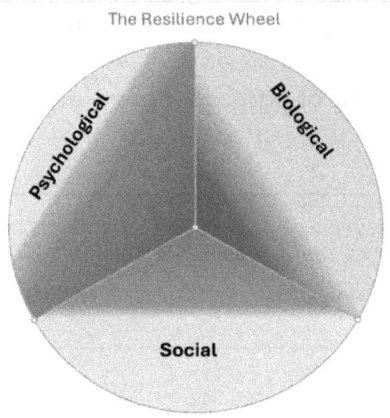

Once you've reflected on your biopsychosocial profile, you'll have a clearer sense of where to focus your energy.

- Are you feeling strong in one pillar but struggling in another? That's a good place to start.
- Do you feel overwhelmed by all three? Focus on the smallest, easiest change in one area—you'll find that progress often builds momentum across other areas too.

In the next section, we'll use this reflection to guide you through setting personalized, actionable goals to strengthen each pillar of resilience and create balance in your life.

SETTING SMART GOALS FOR RESILIENCE

Once you've identified your strengths and challenges in the biopsychosocial pillars, the next step is to turn those insights into actionable goals. Setting goals allows you to focus your energy where it's needed most and track your progress over time. The key is to make your goals personalized, achievable, and aligned with your values.

Your goals will serve as the roadmap for your Resilience Code, helping you take small, meaningful steps toward healing and thriving beyond pain.

SMART goals are an effective way to ensure your efforts are clear and measurable. Each goal should be:

Specific: Clearly define what you want to achieve.

Measurable: Include a way to track your progress.

Achievable: Make sure the goal feels realistic based on your current circumstances.

Relevant: Align your goal with your values and mission.

Time-bound: Set a timeframe to create focus and accountability.

Example SMART Goals by Pillar

Biological Resilience:

- Instead of: "Exercise more."
- Try: "Walk for 10 minutes three times a week for the next month."

Psychological Resilience:

- Instead of: "Be more positive."
- Try: "Write down three things I'm grateful for every evening for the next two weeks."

Social Resilience:

- Instead of: "Reconnect with friends."
- Try: "Call or text one friend each week for the next month to check in and catch up."

How to Choose Goals That Fit Your Life

1. **Start Small**: Focus on one goal per pillar, especially if you feel overwhelmed. Small wins build confidence and momentum.
2. **Align with Your Mission**: Ask yourself how each goal supports your bigger purpose or values.
3. **Be Flexible**: If a goal doesn't work as planned, adjust it. The goal is progress, not perfection.

"What's one small, specific goal I can set for each pillar that feels realistic and meaningful?"

BUILDING BIOLOGICAL RESILIENCE

Biological resilience forms the physical foundation of your Resilience Code. Chronic pain disrupts key systems in your body—your nervous system, immune function, and endocrine balance—leaving you in a constant state of stress and imbalance. Building biological resilience isn't about perfection; it's about creating small, consistent habits that restore balance and help your body work for you instead of against you.

In this section, we'll explore practical strategies to strengthen your biological resilience, from improving sleep and energy to regulating hormones and calming inflammation.

Restoring Nervous System Balance

Your nervous system is the control center for your body, regulating everything from stress responses to pain perception. Chronic pain often keeps the nervous system stuck in "fight or flight" mode, amplifying discomfort and draining energy.

<u>**Key Strategy**</u>

Deep, Restorative Breathing

Why It Works

Breathing techniques like diaphragmatic breathing activate the parasympathetic nervous system, signaling your body to shift into a "rest and repair" state.

How to Do It

Try a 4-7-8 breathing pattern: Inhale for 4 seconds, hold for 7 seconds, and exhale for 8 seconds. Practice for 5–10 minutes daily to calm your system.

Supporting Immune Function and Reducing Inflammation

Chronic pain often creates a cycle of overactive immune responses and systemic inflammation, which can prolong healing and increase sensitivity to pain.

<u>**Key Strategies**</u>

Anti-Inflammatory Nutrition

- Incorporate omega-3 fatty acids (e.g., wild-caught salmon, flaxseeds), colorful fruits, and leafy greens into your diet.
- Minimize inflammatory foods like processed sugars, refined carbohydrates, and excessive alcohol.

Hydration

Stay adequately hydrated to support your body's natural detoxification processes. Use a tracking app or bottle to monitor your intake.

Regulating Endocrine Function

The endocrine system governs key hormones like cortisol, testosterone, and growth hormone, all of which can be disrupted by chronic pain. These imbalances contribute to fatigue, difficulty healing, and emotional instability.

Key Strategies

Strength Training

Resistance exercises help boost testosterone and growth hormone levels while improving overall energy. Start with small, manageable routines like bodyweight exercises or light weights.

Pro Tip

Women also benefit from supporting testosterone levels, which play a crucial role in energy and recovery.

Sleep Hygiene

Establish a consistent sleep routine, limit blue light exposure in the evening, and create a calming bedtime environment.

Why It Works:

Restful sleep is essential for hormone regulation and cellular repair.

Boosting Cellular Energy

Your mitochondria—tiny powerhouses in your cells—are critical for producing the energy your body needs to heal and function. Chronic pain can deplete mitochondrial function, leaving you feeling fatigued.

<u>**Key Strategies**</u>

Zone 2 Exercise

Engage in gentle, aerobic activities (like brisk walking or cycling) that keep your heart rate in a moderate range. This supports mitochondrial health without overtaxing your body.

Studies show that regular Zone 2 aerobic exercise improves mitochondrial function, which is essential for producing the energy your cells need to heal and thrive. This level of exercise—where you can maintain a conversation but still feel challenged—helps your body use oxygen more efficiently, boosting cellular energy without overtaxing your system.

Nutrient Support

Ensure adequate intake of B vitamins, magnesium, and CoQ10, which are vital for energy production.

"Which area of biological resilience—nervous system, immune function, endocrine balance, or energy—feels like the best place for me to start? What's one small change I can make today to support that area?"

STRENGTHENING PSYCHOLOGICAL RESILIENCE

Psychological resilience is the mental and emotional core of your Resilience Code. Chronic pain doesn't just affect your body—it also rewires your brain, creating patterns of fear, stress, and negative thinking that amplify your suffering. Strengthening psychological resilience means reclaiming control of your thoughts and emotions, building new neural pathways, and nurturing a mindset of adaptability and hope.

This section will provide actionable tools to help you reframe negative patterns, manage stress, and cultivate emotional balance.

Reframing Negative Thought Patterns

Chronic pain can lead to cycles of catastrophizing—assuming the worst outcomes—or feeling stuck in helplessness. Breaking these patterns helps reduce the brain's focus on pain.

Key Strategy

Cognitive Reframing

Why It Works

Cognitive reframing trains your brain to challenge and replace negative thoughts with more constructive ones, reducing emotional distress and pain amplification.

How to Do It

- Notice a negative thought (e.g., "I'll never feel better.").
- Challenge it: "Is this thought helpful or true?"
- Reframe it: "I'm working on small changes every day to improve my well-being."

> *"What's one thought I often have about my pain? How can I reframe it to feel more empowered?"*

Managing Stress to Calm the Pain-Stress Cycle

Stress exacerbates pain, and pain creates stress—a vicious cycle. Psychological resilience helps you break this loop by cultivating calm and clarity.

Key Strategies

Progressive Muscle Relaxation (PMR)

Why It Works

PMR reduces tension stored in your body, signaling your brain that it's safe to relax.

How to Do It

Gradually tense and release each muscle group, starting at your feet and working upward.

Heart Coherence Breathing

Why It Works

This technique, supported by research, balances your autonomic nervous system and fosters emotional regulation.

How to Do It

Inhale for 5 seconds, exhale for 5 seconds, and focus on a feeling of gratitude or calm as you breathe.

> *"What's one stress-reduction technique I can try this week? How will I know it's working?"*

Harnessing Neuroplasticity to Rewire the Brain

Your brain is remarkably adaptable. With consistent practice, you can retrain it to focus less on pain and more on positive, meaningful experiences.

<u>Key Strategies</u>

Visualization

Why It Works

Guided imagery and mental rehearsal help create new neural pathways, reducing the brain's focus on pain.

How to Do It

Spend 5–10 minutes visualizing a peaceful place or imagining yourself achieving a goal, engaging all your senses.

Mindfulness Meditation

Why It Works

Meditation increases activity in brain regions associated with calm and emotional regulation while decreasing reactivity in areas like the amygdala.

How to Do It

Start with 5 minutes of focused breathing, observing your thoughts without judgment.

"What's one way I can use visualization or mindfulness to train my brain for resilience?"

BUILDING EMOTIONAL REGULATION SKILLS

Chronic pain often brings emotional turbulence—frustration, sadness, and anger are natural but can feel overwhelming. Psychological resilience helps you navigate these emotions constructively.

Key Strategy

Gratitude Journaling

Why It Works

Gratitude rewires the brain to focus on positive experiences, reducing the emotional toll of pain.

How to Do It

Write down three things you're grateful for each day, focusing on the sensations or emotions they evoke.

"Which area of psychological resilience—thought patterns, stress management, neuroplasticity, or emotional regulation—feels like the best place for me to start? What's one small action I can take today to build resilience in this area?"

ENHANCING SOCIAL RESILIENCE

Social resilience is the connective tissue of your Resilience Code. Chronic pain often isolates you, straining relationships and cutting you off from vital sources of support. Yet, meaningful connection is one of the most powerful tools for healing—it reduces stress, enhances emotional well-being, and even impacts your biology by releasing oxytocin, the "bonding hormone."

In this section, we'll explore practical strategies to rebuild trust, foster connection, and create a network of support that uplifts and sustains you.

Rebuilding Trust and Connection

Pain can strain relationships, leading to misunderstandings or withdrawal. Rebuilding trust starts with small, consistent actions and open communication.

Key Strategies

Honest Conversations

Why It Works

Expressing your needs and limitations helps others understand your experience and find ways to support you.

How to Do It

Start with simple, clear statements like: "I want to spend time with you, but I may need to leave early if my pain flares up."

Quality Over Quantity

Why It Works

Focus on nurturing a few meaningful relationships rather than spreading yourself thin.

Positive social interactions, such as open, empathetic conversations, have been shown to release oxytocin, the "bonding hormone." Oxytocin not only fosters emotional connection but also reduces stress hormones like cortisol, creating a sense of safety and stability. These biological effects make trust and connection powerful tools for resilience.

"What's one relationship I value that could benefit from an open, honest conversation?"

Finding New Sources of Support

Sometimes your existing network isn't enough, and that's okay. Building new connections can open doors to support and understanding you didn't know were possible.

Key Strategies

Explore Online Communities

Why It Works

Safe, supportive online spaces allow you to connect with people who share similar challenges without the pressure of in-person interactions.

Pro Tip

Look for groups with clear guidelines for respect and active moderation to ensure a positive experience.

Join Local Activities

Why It Works

Community classes or volunteer opportunities can help you meet new people while pursuing interests that align with your values.

"What's one new community or activity I could explore to expand my support network?"

Strengthening Bonds with Small Gestures

Connection doesn't always require grand actions. Small, thoughtful gestures can deepen relationships and foster a sense of belonging.

Key Strategies

Gratitude in Action

Why It Works

Expressing appreciation strengthens emotional bonds and boosts oxytocin levels.

How to Do It

Write a heartfelt thank-you note or send a simple text letting someone know you appreciate them.

Shared Rituals

Why It Works

Creating rituals—like weekly coffee chats or family dinners—reinforces connection and provides a consistent source of joy.

"What's one small gesture I could make this week to show someone I care?"

Setting Boundaries for Healthy Relationships

Protecting your energy is essential, especially when some relationships feel draining or unsupportive. Setting boundaries allows you to prioritize connections that uplift you.

Key Strategies

Learn to Say No with Kindness

Why It Works

Saying no to what doesn't serve you creates space for what does.

How to Do It

Use statements like: "I'd love to help, but I'm at my limit right now."

Focus on Mutual Support

Why It Works

Healthy relationships are balanced, with give-and-take that leaves both people feeling valued.

> *"Which area of social resilience—rebuilding trust, finding support, small gestures, or setting boundaries—feels like the best place for me to start? What's one small action I can take today to strengthen my connections?"*

TRACKING YOUR PROGRESS

To stay motivated, it's important to track your efforts and celebrate your wins, no matter how small. Tools like habit trackers, apps, or journals can help you stay on course.

How Long Does It Take to Build a Habit?

You may have heard that it takes 28 days to form a habit, but research tells a more nuanced story. A 2009 study published in the *European Journal of Social Psychology* found that it takes on average about 66 days for a habit to feel automatic. However, the time frame varies significantly—some habits take as little as 18 days, while others may require up to 254 days, depending on the complexity of the behavior and individual circumstances.

The key to forming habits isn't perfection—it's consistency over time. Even if you miss a day or two, that doesn't mean you've failed. Building a habit is about steady progress, not an unbroken streak. Focus on small, consistent actions that align with your goals, and allow yourself the flexibility to adapt as needed.

Consistently practicing habits like gratitude or mindfulness strengthens neural pathways associated with positive thinking and emotional regulation. Research shows that over time, these practices can reduce the brain's focus on pain signals and increase activity in areas linked to calm and resilience.

Simple Tracking Methods

- Use a calendar to check off days when you complete your goal.

- Write a weekly reflection about what went well and what could improve.
- Try an app like Strides or Streaks to gamify your progress.

"What's one way I can make tracking my progress enjoyable and motivating?"

TRACKING YOUR PROGRESS AND ADAPTING OVER TIME

Resilience isn't a linear journey—it's a dynamic process. Life's challenges, changing circumstances, and even progress itself can shift your needs and priorities. That's why your Resilience Code isn't static—it's a living framework designed to evolve with you.

In this section, we'll explore how to regularly assess your progress through resilience check-ins, adapt your plan as needed, and celebrate your wins along the way. Flexibility is the key to maintaining momentum while ensuring your goals remain aligned with your life.

How to Conduct a Resilience Check-In

Regular resilience check-ins give you a structured way to evaluate how you're doing and adjust your focus as needed.

1. **Schedule Your Check-Ins**:
    - Choose a consistent timeframe—weekly, biweekly, or monthly.
    - Block off 15–30 minutes to reflect on your progress and challenges.
2. **Ask Key Questions**:
    - Biological Resilience: "Am I feeling more energized and physically capable?"
    - Psychological Resilience: "Am I handling stress and emotions better?"

- Social Resilience: "Am I feeling supported and connected?"
- Overall: "What's working well, and what needs to change?"

3. **Bring in Trusted Feedback**:
    - Invite a trusted social support (e.g., a partner, friend, or mentor) to share their observations.
    - Ask questions like:
        - "Do you notice changes in how I'm managing stress or engaging with others?"
        - "What progress have you seen in me that I might not recognize myself?"

Bringing in external feedback provides an objective perspective, helping you identify blind spots and celebrate achievements you may overlook.

Adapting Your Plan

If something isn't working, that's okay—adaptation is part of the process.

- **Refine Your Goals**
    - If a goal feels too difficult, break it into smaller steps.
    - If a goal feels too easy, challenge yourself to level up.
- **Reassess Priorities**:
    - Sometimes, life shifts, and what felt urgent last month may no longer be a priority. Adjust your focus to match your current needs.
- **Revisit the Biopsychosocial Framework**:
    - Use the **Resilience Wheel** to visualize changes in your strengths and weaknesses. For example, if you've made great strides socially but feel stalled biologically, shift focus accordingly.

Setbacks are a natural part of any journey, and resilience means learning to adapt rather than giving up. When you face a challenge or a missed goal, take a moment to reflect:

- What might have contributed to the setback?
- What's one small adjustment I can make to regain momentum?

Remember, progress isn't linear—it's about staying flexible and committed to your mission, even when the road gets bumpy.

Celebrate Small Wins

Progress deserves recognition, no matter how small. Celebrating your successes reinforces positive change and keeps you motivated.

Create Milestones: Treat yourself when you reach a milestone, like completing a week of daily movement or reconnecting with a loved one.

Reflect on Your Growth: Journaling or sharing your progress with a trusted friend can make your achievements feel more tangible.

"What's one small win I've had recently, and how can I celebrate it in a way that feels meaningful?"

By conducting regular resilience check-ins and involving trusted supports when needed, you'll ensure your plan remains flexible and effective. Tracking and adapting your Resilience Code allows it to grow with you, evolving into a powerful tool for long-term healing and thriving. In the next section, we'll discuss how to reclaim your mission and align your actions with the purpose and values that matter most to you.

RECLAIMING YOUR MISSION

Chronic pain is an unfortunate and often deeply challenging part of life. But pain doesn't have to define you—it can refine you.

Just as a cocoon creates the conditions for transformation, pain can serve as the crucible that shapes who you are meant to be. While no one chooses this path, it can lead to a new sense of purpose, one that aligns with your strengths, values, and resilience.

Reclaiming your mission isn't about going back to who you were before the pain. It's about stepping into who you are now and who you're meant to become. True resilience isn't just about enduring challenges—it's about using them to create something new and meaningful.

In this chapter, we'll explore how the cocoon of pain, while difficult, can give rise to a metamorphosis—a redirection of purpose and identity that aligns with your values and strengths. This is the essence of the Peak Resilience Method: turning adversity into a foundation for growth, fulfillment, and thriving.

Zooming Out: Redefining Your Mission

Sometimes, pain forces you to let go of specific goals or activities that once felt central to your identity. But the core of your mission—your deeper "why"—remains intact. It may just need to be reframed or expressed in new ways.

For example:

- If you saw yourself as an athlete but can no longer participate in high-impact sports, your mission might shift to inspiring others to find joy in movement, whether through coaching, writing, or community fitness initiatives.
- If your mission was rooted in creativity, like painting or music, but chronic pain limits your physical abilities, it might expand into teaching, mentoring, or advocating for access to the arts.

This reframing builds on the idea of flexibility and adaptability we explored in earlier chapters. It's not about abandoning your passions—it's about finding new ways to honor them.

"What deeper values or meaning lie at the heart of the things I once loved to do? How could I honor those values in new ways?"

Aligning Your Resilience Code with Your Mission

You've seen these pillars before, but we're highlighting them here because they form the foundation for reclaiming your mission. Start by identifying one goal from each pillar that aligns with your mission. For example:

Biological: Improving your energy levels so you can volunteer weekly.

Psychological: Building confidence in your ability to reframe negative thoughts about setbacks.

Social: Strengthening your relationships to create a network of support as you pursue your mission.

Let's look at how this might work in practice:

Biological: A teacher with chronic fatigue focuses on improving energy through better hydration and consistent sleep hygiene, allowing them to stay engaged with their students.

Psychological: A musician uses visualization techniques to overcome self-doubt before performances, rediscovering their joy in sharing music.

Social: A caregiver strengthens their network by joining a local support group, finding encouragement and practical advice to balance their role and personal needs.

> *"What's one action you can take today that feels meaningful and brings you closer to the life you envision?"*

Bringing Others into Your Mission

Sharing your mission with others can amplify its impact and inspire collaboration. Involve trusted friends, family, or community members in your goals to create accountability and shared purpose.

- Share your mission with a friend and ask for their support in brainstorming ideas or celebrating milestones.
- Create traditions or rituals that reflect your mission, like volunteering together or hosting gatherings that bring people together around your shared values.

Research has shown that oxytocin, often called the "bonding hormone," plays a significant role in reducing stress and fostering feelings of trust and connection. Positive social interactions, like sharing laughter or a kind gesture, stimulate oxytocin release, helping to calm the nervous system and lower cortisol levels. Studies have also suggested that oxytocin may enhance resilience by promoting cooperation and emotional stability.

> *"Who in my life can I share my mission with, and how can we work together to bring it to life?"*

Aligning your life with your mission doesn't just impact you—it creates a ripple effect that spreads healing, connection, and inspiration to others. While we've touched on this idea before, it's worth repeating: the work you do to reclaim your life has a powerful, far-reaching influence.

For instance, one reader shared their newfound mission of

mentoring local youth. This not only reignited their sense of purpose but also inspired others in their community to step forward and volunteer. The ripple effect of one person's resilience and commitment can spark change far beyond what they initially imagined.

"What legacy do I want my mission to leave behind? How can I take one step toward that vision today?"

Here's what thriving looks like when resilience becomes a way of life:

- **Biologically**: You listen to your body, honor its needs, and make choices that support your energy and health.
- **Psychologically**: You approach stress with curiosity and flexibility, knowing that setbacks are opportunities for growth.
- **Socially**: You nurture relationships that uplift and sustain you, while also setting boundaries that protect your well-being.

When resilience becomes second nature, your mission can take center stage.

Your mission doesn't have to be grand or world-changing; it just needs to reflect what gives your life meaning.

Living in alignment with your mission means making choices, big and small, that support the values you hold most dear.

For example, if connection is one of your core values, you might set aside 15 minutes each day to call a loved one, send a thoughtful message, or schedule time to meet with a friend. If creativity is central to your mission, you could dedicate time to brainstorming projects, taking a class, or teaching others your craft. Small actions that reflect your values can ripple out to create meaningful change over time.

"What's one small decision I can make today that aligns with my mission and values?"

THRIVING THROUGH FUTURE CHALLENGES

The tools and habits you've built throughout this journey don't just help you recover from chronic pain—they prepare you for life's inevitable ups and downs. Challenges will still arise, but your resilience will help you face them with confidence and adaptability.

Practical Strategies for Maintaining Resilience:

- **Revisit Your Resilience Code**: Periodically assess your goals and adjust them to reflect where you are now.
- **Build a Resilience Routine**: Incorporate daily practices like mindfulness, gratitude, or movement that keep you grounded.
- **Lean on Your Support Network**: Stay connected to the people and communities that help you thrive.

"How can I use the lessons I've learned to face future challenges with strength and clarity?"

CONCLUSION: THIS IS JUST THE BEGINNING

This journey has been about more than chronic pain—it's been about rediscovering your capacity to adapt, heal, and thrive. The tools you've gained are now yours to carry forward, not just to address pain but to navigate whatever challenges life may bring.

Like Sarah, you now have the tools to reclaim your mission and move forward with resilience. Her journey from pain to purpose is proof that small, intentional steps can lead to profound transformation.

You have everything you need to create your own story of thriving, no matter the challenges you face.

As you move forward, remember that resilience isn't something you achieve once—it's a practice you cultivate every day. With your Resilience Code as your guide, you have the framework to build the life you want, one step at a time.

Like a butterfly emerging from its cocoon, you are stepping into a life of resilience and purpose. The challenges you've faced have shaped you into someone stronger, more adaptable, and ready to thrive. With your Resilience Code as your guide, you're prepared to embrace life's possibilities and write the next chapter of your story.

Affirmation: *I have the strength to integrate the tools I've learned. Each step I take—no matter how small—brings me closer to a life of resilience, purpose, and wellness.*

BIBLIOGRAPHY

INTRODUCTION

1. Felitti, V. J., Anda, R. F., Nordenberg, D., Williamson, D. F., Spitz, A. M., Edwards, V., & Marks, J. S. (1998). Relationship of childhood abuse and household dysfunction to many of the leading causes of death in adults: The Adverse Childhood Experiences (ACE) study. *American Journal of Preventive Medicine, 14*(4), 245–258. https://doi.org/10.1016/S0749-3797(98)00017-8
2. Kabat-Zinn, J. (1990). *Full catastrophe living: Using the wisdom of your body and mind to face stress, pain, and illness.* Delacorte Press.
3. Moseley, G. L., & Butler, D. S. (2015). *Explain pain supercharged.* Noigroup Publications.
4. Chrousos, G. P. (1995). The hypothalamic-pituitary-adrenal axis and immune-mediated inflammation. *New England Journal of Medicine, 332*(20), 1351–1362. https://doi.org/10.1056/NEJM199505183322008
5. Panksepp, J. (2003). Neuroscience. Social bonding: Emotional roots of love and prosocial behavior. *Current Directions in Psychological Science, 11*(6), 259–263. https://doi.org/10.1111/1467-8721.00147

CHAPTER ONE

1. Chrousos, G. P. (1995). The hypothalamic-pituitary-adrenal axis and immune-mediated inflammation. *New England Journal of Medicine, 332*(20), 1351–1362. https://doi.org/10.1056/NEJM199505183322008 (Referenced for stress responses and their impact on chronic pain).
2. Moseley, G. L., & Butler, D. S. (2015). *Explain Pain Supercharged.* Noigroup Publications. (Utilized for understanding chronic pain's impact on the brain and neuroplasticity).
3. Felitti, V. J., Anda, R. F., Nordenberg, D., Williamson, D. F., Spitz, A. M., Edwards, V., & Marks, J. S. (1998). Relationship of childhood abuse and household dysfunction to many of the leading causes of death in adults: The Adverse Childhood Experiences (ACE) study. *American Journal of Preventive Medicine, 14*(4), 245–258. https://doi.org/10.1016/S0749-3797(98)00017-8 (Cited for its foundational insights on ACEs and their long-term health impacts).

BIBLIOGRAPHY

4. Felitti, V. J., Anda, R. F., Nordenberg, D., Williamson, D. F., Spitz, A. M., Edwards, V., & Marks, J. S. (1998). Relationship of childhood abuse and household dysfunction to many of the leading causes of death in adults: The Adverse Childhood Experiences (ACE) study. *American Journal of Preventive Medicine, 14*(4), 245–258. https://doi.org/10.1016/S0749-3797(98)00017-8:contentReference{index=0}.
5. Moseley, G. L., & Butler, D. S. (2015). *Explain pain supercharged*. Noigroup Publications. (Referenced for understanding chronic pain pathways and the role of biopsychosocial factors).
6. Kabat-Zinn, J. (1990). *Full catastrophe living: Using the wisdom of your body and mind to face stress, pain, and illness.* Delacorte Press. (Referenced for mindfulness practices related to pain resilience).

CHAPTERS TWO AND THREE

1. Kabat-Zinn, J. (1990). *Full catastrophe living: Using the wisdom of your body and mind to face stress, pain, and illness.* Delacorte Press. (Referenced for mindfulness practices and their effect on resilience).
2. Felitti, V. J., Anda, R. F., Nordenberg, D., Williamson, D. F., Spitz, A. M., Edwards, V., & Marks, J. S. (1998). Relationship of childhood abuse and household dysfunction to many of the leading causes of death in adults: The Adverse Childhood Experiences (ACE) study. *American Journal of Preventive Medicine, 14*(4), 245–258. https://doi.org/10.1016/S0749-3797(98)00017-8. (Cited for insights into early trauma's role in chronic pain resilience).
3. Moseley, G. L., & Butler, D. S. (2015). *Explain pain supercharged*. Noigroup Publications. (Referenced for its examination of chronic pain pathways and their neuroplasticity).
4. Siegel, D. J. (2010). *The mindful therapist: A clinician's guide to mindsight and neural integration.* W.W. Norton & Company. (Referenced for understanding emotional regulation and its contribution to psychological resilience).

CHAPTERS FOUR AND FIVE

1. Barati, K., & Rahimdel, A. (2019). Mitochondrial dysfunction in osteoarthritis: A systematic review. *Journal of Translational Medicine, 17*(1), 87. https://doi.org/10.1186/s12967-019-1864-y. (Cited for insights into mitochondrial dysfunction and chronic pain management).
2. Khalid, A., & Dong, W. (2019). Antioxidants in neuropathic pain treatment: Role of CoQ10 and alpha-lipoic acid in ROS reduction. *Antioxidants, 8*(7), 238. https://doi.org/10.3390/

antiox8070238. (Referenced for the role of CoQ10 and alpha-lipoic acid in mitochondrial efficiency and oxidative stress).

3. Fasano, A., & Shea-Donohue, T. (2005). Mechanisms of disease: The role of intestinal barrier function in the pathogenesis of gastrointestinal autoimmune diseases. *Nature Clinical Practice Gastroenterology & Hepatology, 2*(9), 416–422. https://doi.org/10.1038/ncpgasthep0259. (Referenced for understanding the gut-brain axis and its role in inflammation).

4. Chrousos, G. P. (1995). The hypothalamic-pituitary-adrenal axis and immune-mediated inflammation. *New England Journal of Medicine, 332*(20), 1351–1362. https://doi.org/10.1056/NEJM199505183322008. (Cited for chronic pain mechanisms and the HPA axis).

5. Kabat-Zinn, J. (1990). *Full catastrophe living: Using the wisdom of your body and mind to face stress, pain, and illness.* Delacorte Press. (Referenced for resilience practices such as mindfulness in chronic pain management).

6. Chrousos, G. P. (1995). The hypothalamic-pituitary-adrenal axis and immune-mediated inflammation. *New England Journal of Medicine, 332*(20), 1351–1362. https://doi.org/10.1056/NEJM199505183322008. (Discussed for its insights on stress, hormonal changes, and their impact on chronic pain resilience).

7. Fasano, A., & Shea-Donohue, T. (2005). Mechanisms of disease: The role of intestinal barrier function in the pathogenesis of gastrointestinal autoimmune diseases. *Nature Clinical Practice Gastroenterology & Hepatology, 2*(9), 416–422. https://doi.org/10.1038/ncpgasthep0259. (Referenced for gut health and its influence on inflammation).

8. Kabat-Zinn, J. (1990). *Full catastrophe living: Using the wisdom of your body and mind to face stress, pain, and illness.* Delacorte Press. (Referenced for the integration of mindfulness in chronic pain management).

9. Selye, H. (1956). *The Stress of Life.* McGraw-Hill. (Referenced for the foundational concepts of stress adaptation and resilience).

CHAPTERS SIX AND SEVEN

1. Kabat-Zinn, J. (1990). *Full catastrophe living: Using the wisdom of your body and mind to face stress, pain, and illness.* Delacorte Press. (Referenced for mindfulness strategies to calm the mind and manage chronic pain).

2. Moseley, G. L., & Butler, D. S. (2015). *Explain pain supercharged.* Noigroup Publications. (Referenced for insights on neuroplasticity and chronic pain pathways).

3. Chrousos, G. P. (1995). The hypothalamic-pituitary-adrenal axis and immune-mediated inflammation. *New England Journal of Medicine, 332*(20), 1351–1362. https://doi.org/10.1056/NEJM199505183322008.

BIBLIOGRAPHY

(Referenced for the physiological impacts of stress on the nervous system and inflammation).

4. Apkarian, A. V., Baliki, M. N., & Geha, P. Y. "Towards a Theory of Chronic Pain." *Progress in Neurobiology* 87, no. 2 (2009): 81-97. https://doi.org/10.1016/j.pneurobio.2008.09.018.

5. Baliki, M. N., Geha, P. Y., Apkarian, A. V., & Chialvo, D. R. "Beyond Feeling: Chronic Pain Hurts the Brain, Disrupting the Default-Mode Network Dynamics." *The Journal of Neuroscience* 28, no. 6 (2008): 1398-1403. https://doi.org/10.1523/JNEUROSCI.4123-07.2008.

6. Bushnell, M. C., Čeko, M., & Low, L. A. "Cognitive and Emotional Control of Pain and Its Disruption in Chronic Pain." *Nature Reviews Neuroscience* 14, no. 7 (2013): 502-511. https://doi.org/10.1038/nrn3516.

7. Garland, E. L., Pain, T., Priddy, S. E., & Howard, M. O. "Mindfulness-Oriented Recovery Enhancement for Chronic Pain and Prescription Opioid Misuse: Results from an Early-Stage Randomized Controlled Trial." *Journal of Consulting and Clinical Psychology* 82, no. 3 (2014): 448-459. https://doi.org/10.1037/a0035798.

8. Goyal, M., Singh, S., Sibinga, E. M. S., et al. "Meditation Programs for Psychological Stress and Well-Being: A Systematic Review and Meta-Analysis." *JAMA Internal Medicine* 174, no. 3 (2014): 357-368. https://doi.org/10.1001/jamainternmed.2013.13018.

9. Seminowicz, D. A., & Moayedi, M. "The Dorsolateral Prefrontal Cortex in Acute and Chronic Pain." *The Journal of Pain* 18, no. 9 (2017): 1027-1035. https://doi.org/10.1016/j.jpain.2017.03.008.

10. Zeidan, F., Martucci, K. T., Kraft, R. A., Gordon, N. S., McHaffie, J. G., & Coghill, R. C. "Brain Mechanisms Supporting the Modulation of Pain by Mindfulness Meditation." *The Journal of Neuroscience* 31, no. 14 (2011): 5540-5548. https://doi.org/10.1523/JNEUROSCI.5791-10.2011.

11. Wright, Robert. *Why Buddhism Is True: The Science and Philosophy of Meditation and Enlightenment.* New York: Simon & Schuster, 2017.

CHAPTER EIGHT

1. Felitti, V. J., Anda, R. F., Nordenberg, D., Williamson, D. F., Spitz, A. M., Edwards, V., & Marks, J. S. (1998). Relationship of childhood abuse and household dysfunction to many of the leading causes of death in adults: The Adverse Childhood Experiences (ACE) study. *American Journal of Preventive Medicine, 14*(4), 245–258. https://doi.org/10.1016/S0749-3797(98)00017-8. (Referenced for understanding the connection between early trauma and chronic health issues).

2. Kabat-Zinn, J. (1990). *Full catastrophe living: Using the wisdom of your body and mind to face stress, pain, and illness.* Delacorte Press. (Discussed for mindfulness practices aiding trauma recovery).

3. Porges, S. W. (2009). The polyvagal theory: New insights into adaptive reactions of the autonomic nervous system. *Cleveland Clinic Journal of Medicine, 76*(2), S86–S90. https://doi.org/10.3949/ccjm.76.s2.17. (Explored for understanding trauma's effects on the nervous system).
4. van der Kolk, B. A. (2014). *The body keeps the score: Brain, mind, and body in the healing of trauma*. Viking Penguin. (Referenced for insights into how trauma rewires the brain and its implications for chronic pain).

CHAPTER NINE

Social Connection, Pain Perception, and Resilience

1. Panksepp, Jaak. "Neuroscience. Social Bonding: Emotional Roots of Love and Prosocial Behavior." *Current Directions in Psychological Science* 11, no. 6 (2003): 259–63. https://doi.org/10.1111/1467-8721.00147.
2. → *Discusses how social bonding reduces pain perception and promotes resilience.*
3. Rat Park Experiment (1978). Alexander, Bruce K., Robert B. Coambs, and Patricia F. Hadaway. "The Effect of Housing and Gender on Morphine Self-Administration in Rats." *Psychopharmacology* 58, no. 2 (1978): 175–79. https://doi.org/10.1007/BF00426903.
4. → *Provides insight into how social environments influence stress and addiction, relevant to social resilience in chronic pain.*
5. Kabat-Zinn, Jon. *Full Catastrophe Living: Using the Wisdom of Your Body and Mind to Face Stress, Pain, and Illness.* New York: Delacorte Press, 1990.
6. → *Referenced for mindfulness-based strategies to reduce social isolation and manage chronic pain.*
7. Moseley, G. Lorimer, and David S. Butler. *Explain Pain Supercharged.* Adelaide, Australia: Noigroup Publications, 2015.
8. → *Explores the interplay between social connection and pain perception.*

Neuroscience of Social Isolation, Stress, and Pain

1. Eisenberger, Naomi I., and Matthew D. Lieberman. "Why It Hurts to Be Left Out: The Neurocognitive Overlap Between Physical and Social Pain." *Trends in Cognitive Sciences* 8, no. 7 (2004): 294–300. https://doi.org/10.1016/j.tics.2004.05.010.
2. → *Discusses how the brain processes social rejection similarly to physical pain.*
3. Cacioppo, John T., and Louise C. Hawkley. "Perceived Social Isolation and Cognition." *Trends in Cognitive Sciences* 13, no. 10 (2009): 447–54. https://doi.org/10.1016/j.tics.2009.06.005.
4. → *Explains the physiological and cognitive consequences of social disconnection, including increased inflammation and pain sensitivity.*

BIBLIOGRAPHY

5. Carter, Sue, Stephen W. Porges, and Mary S. Barchas. "Neuropeptides and the Social Brain: Oxytocin and Vasopressin in the Regulation of Social Behaviors." *Frontiers in Neuroendocrinology* 32, no. 4 (2011): 251–74. https://doi.org/10.1016/j.yfrne.2011.07.001.
6. → *Discusses oxytocin's role in buffering stress and pain, supporting the chapter's section on how social connection reduces neuroinflammation.*
7. Slavich, George M., and Steven W. Cole. "The Emerging Field of Human Social Genomics." *Clinical Psychological Science* 1, no. 3 (2013): 331–48. https://doi.org/10.1177/2167702613478594.
8. → *Explores how social isolation increases pro-inflammatory gene expression, worsening chronic pain symptoms.*

ME/CFS, Fibromyalgia, and Hidden Pain

1. Komaroff, Anthony L., and José G. Lipkin. "Insights from Advances in Research on Chronic Fatigue Syndrome and Myalgic Encephalomyelitis." *JAMA* 322, no. 6 (2019): 499–500. https://doi.org/10.1001/jama.2019.8312.
2. → *Provides scientific evidence on ME/CFS as a legitimate biomedical condition, countering stigma surrounding the disease.*
3. Jason, Leonard A., and Abigail Brown. "Stigma and Chronic Fatigue Syndrome: A Review of the Literature." *Stigma and Health* 2, no. 4 (2017): 282–92. https://doi.org/10.1037/sah0000055.
4. → *Discusses how societal attitudes toward ME/CFS contribute to isolation and reinforce cycles of distress.*
5. Clauw, Daniel J. "Fibromyalgia: A Clinical Review." *JAMA* 311, no. 15 (2014): 1547–55. https://doi.org/10.1001/jama.2014.3266.
6. → *Explains the neurological mechanisms of fibromyalgia, its lack of clear diagnostic markers, and why it is often misunderstood.*
7. Kindlon, Tom. "Post-Exertional Malaise in Myalgic Encephalomyelitis/Chronic Fatigue Syndrome." *Healthcare* 8, no. 4 (2020): 211. https://doi.org/10.3390/healthcare8040211.
8. → *Describes the post-exertional malaise component of ME/CFS, reinforcing Raj's narrative struggles with unpredictable energy crashes.*

Additional Sources on Chronic Pain, Stigma, and Psychological Resilience

1. Williams, Amanda C. de C., and Kevin G. E. Geddes. "Cognitive Behavioral Therapy for Chronic Pain: An Overview." *British Journal of Pain* 11, no. 2 (2017): 55–64. https://doi.org/10.1177/2049463717696676.
2. → *Explains the role of cognitive reframing in shifting negative pain-related thought patterns and reducing distress.*

3. Sharpe, Michael, et al. "A Biopsychosocial Approach to Chronic Pain: Beyond the 'Medicate or Operate' Model." *BMJ* 357 (2017): j1996. https://doi.org/10.1136/bmj.j1996.
4. → *Supports the chapter's argument for addressing chronic pain through social, psychological, and biological factors.*

CHAPTER TEN

1. Alexander, Bruce K., Robert B. Coambs, and Patricia F. Hadaway. "The Effect of Housing and Gender on Morphine Self-Administration in Rats." *Psychopharmacology* 58, no. 2 (1978): 175–179. https://doi.org/10.1007/BF00426903.
2. Cacioppo, John T., and William Patrick. *Loneliness: Human Nature and the Need for Social Connection.* New York: W. W. Norton & Company, 2008.
3. Carter, Sue C. "Neuroendocrine Perspectives on Social Attachment and Love." *Psychoneuroendocrinology* 23, no. 8 (1998): 779–818. https://doi.org/10.1016/S0306-4530(98)00055-9.
4. Eisenberger, Naomi I., and Matthew D. Lieberman. "Why Rejection Hurts: A Common Neural Alarm System for Physical and Social Pain." *Trends in Cognitive Sciences* 9, no. 7 (2005): 294–300. https://doi.org/10.1016/j.tics.2005.05.010.
5. Kabat-Zinn, Jon. *Full Catastrophe Living: Using the Wisdom of Your Body and Mind to Face Stress, Pain, and Illness.* New York: Delacorte Press, 1990.
6. Moseley, G. Lorimer, and David S. Butler. *Explain Pain Supercharged.* Adelaide: Noigroup Publications, 2015.
7. Panksepp, Jaak. "Neuroscience. Social Bonding: Emotional Roots of Love and Prosocial Behavior." *Current Directions in Psychological Science* 11, no. 6 (2003): 259–263. https://doi.org/10.1111/1467-8721.00147.
8. Slavich, George M., and Steve W. Cole. "The Emerging Field of Human Social Genomics." *Clinical Psychological Science* 1, no. 3 (2013): 331–348. https://doi.org/10.1177/2167702613478594.
9. Van Heukelom, Rik, et al. "The Impact of Loneliness on Pain Perception and the Role of Social Support." *Pain Reports* 5, no. 6 (2020): e851. https://doi.org/10.1097/PR9.0000000000000851.
10. Harvard Study of Adult Development. "The Key to Living a Happy Life." *Harvard Gazette,* April 11, 2017. https://news.harvard.edu/gazette/story/2017/04/over-nearly-80-years-harvard-study-has-been-showing-how-to-live-a-healthy-and-happy-life/.

BIBLIOGRAPHY

CHAPTER ELEVEN

1. Kabat-Zinn, J. (1990). *Full catastrophe living: Using the wisdom of your body and mind to face stress, pain, and illness.* Delacorte Press. (Referenced for mindfulness practices in managing pain cycles and amplifiers).
2. Moseley, G. L., & Butler, D. S. (2015). *Explain pain supercharged.* Noigroup Publications. (Cited for understanding feedback loops in chronic pain and the role of neuroplasticity).
3. van der Kolk, B. A. (2014). *The body keeps the score: Brain, mind, and body in the healing of trauma.* Penguin Books. (Referenced for the interplay between psychological and physiological amplifiers).
4. Chrousos, G. P. (1995). The hypothalamic-pituitary-adrenal axis and immune-mediated inflammation. *New England Journal of Medicine, 332*(20), 1351–1362. https://doi.org/10.1056/NEJM199505183322008. (Discussed for its explanation of stress responses in amplifying pain).

CHAPTER TWELVE

1. Felitti, V. J., Anda, R. F., Nordenberg, D., Williamson, D. F., Spitz, A. M., Edwards, V., & Marks, J. S. (1998). Relationship of childhood abuse and household dysfunction to many of the leading causes of death in adults: The Adverse Childhood Experiences (ACE) study. *American Journal of Preventive Medicine, 14*(4), 245–258. https://doi.org/10.1016/S0749-3797(98)00017-8. (Referenced for understanding the connection between early trauma and chronic health issues).
2. Kabat-Zinn, J. (1990). *Full catastrophe living: Using the wisdom of your body and mind to face stress, pain, and illness.* Delacorte Press. (Discussed for mindfulness practices aiding trauma recovery).
3. Porges, S. W. (2009). The polyvagal theory: New insights into adaptive reactions of the autonomic nervous system. *Cleveland Clinic Journal of Medicine, 76*(2), S86–S90. https://doi.org/10.3949/ccjm.76.s2.17. (Explored for understanding trauma's effects on the nervous system).
4. van der Kolk, B. A. (2014). *The body keeps the score: Brain, mind, and body in the healing of trauma.* Viking Penguin. (Referenced for insights into how trauma rewires the brain and its implications for chronic pain).

CHAPTER THIRTEEN

1. Barati, K., & Rahimdel, A. (2019). Mitochondrial dysfunction in osteoarthritis: A systematic review. *Journal of Translational Medicine, 17*(1), 87. https://doi.org/10.1186/s12967-019-1864-y. (Discussed for insights into mitochondrial health and energy restoration).

2. Khalid, A., & Dong, W. (2019). Antioxidants in neuropathic pain treatment: Role of CoQ10 and alpha-lipoic acid in ROS reduction. *Antioxidants, 8*(7), 238. https://doi.org/10.3390/antiox8070238. (Referenced for the role of antioxidants in reducing inflammation and improving cellular health).
3. Kabat-Zinn, J. (1990). *Full catastrophe living: Using the wisdom of your body and mind to face stress, pain, and illness.* Delacorte Press. (Referenced for strategies to manage chronic stress and support endocrine balance).
4. Selye, H. (1956). *The Stress of Life.* McGraw-Hill. (Utilized for foundational insights into how stress impacts the endocrine system and overall resilience).
5. Moseley, G. L., & Butler, D. S. (2015). *Explain pain supercharged.* Noigroup Publications. (Explored for its discussion of pain pathways and their regulation through biological resilience practices).

CHAPTER FOURTEEN

1. Kabat-Zinn, J. (1990). *Full catastrophe living: Using the wisdom of your body and mind to face stress, pain, and illness.* Delacorte Press. (Referenced for mindfulness practices and their role in psychological resilience).
2. Moseley, G. L., & Butler, D. S. (2015). *Explain pain supercharged.* Noigroup Publications. (Discussed for the relationship between neuroplasticity and chronic pain).
3. Siegel, D. J. (2010). *The mindful therapist: A clinician's guide to mindsight and neural integration.* W.W. Norton & Company. (Explored for its insights on building emotional resilience through mindfulness and self-regulation).
4. van der Kolk, B. A. (2014). *The body keeps the score: Brain, mind, and body in the healing of trauma.* Viking Penguin. (Referenced for understanding trauma's impact on the brain and its relevance to chronic pain recovery).

CHAPTER FIFTEEN

1. Alexander, B. K., Coambs, R. B., & Hadaway, P. F. (1978). The effect of housing and gender on morphine self-administration in rats. *Psychopharmacology, 58*(2), 175–179. https://doi.org/10.1007/BF00426903. (Referenced for the Rat Park experiment, illustrating the power of social connection in reducing stress and substance dependence).
2. Panksepp, J. (2003). Neuroscience. Social bonding: Emotional roots of love and prosocial behavior. *Current Directions in Psychological Science, 11*(6), 259–263. https://doi.org/10.1111/1467-8721.00147. (Discussed for the biological impact of social connections, including oxytocin's role in calming the nervous system).

BIBLIOGRAPHY

3. Siegel, D. J. (2010). *The mindful therapist: A clinician's guide to mindsight and neural integration.* W.W. Norton & Company. (Explored for insights into building healthier interpersonal relationships through mindfulness).
4. van der Kolk, B. A. (2014). *The body keeps the score: Brain, mind, and body in the healing of trauma.* Viking Penguin. (Referenced for understanding the interplay between trauma and disrupted social relationships).

CHAPTER SIXTEEN

1. Crum, A. J., Salovey, P., & Achor, S. (2013). Rethinking stress: The role of mindsets in determining the stress response. *Journal of Personality and Social Psychology, 104*(4), 716–733. https://doi.org/10.1037/a0031201
2. Henningsen, P., Zipfel, S., & Herzog, W. (2007). Management of functional somatic syndromes. *The Lancet, 369*(9565), 946–955. https://doi.org/10.1016/S0140-6736(07)60159-7
3. Kabat-Zinn, J. (1990). *Full catastrophe living: Using the wisdom of your body and mind to face stress, pain, and illness.* Delta.
4. LeDoux, J. E. (2000). Emotion circuits in the brain. *Annual Review of Neuroscience, 23*(1), 155–184. https://doi.org/10.1146/annurev.neuro.23.1.155
5. Melzack, R., & Wall, P. D. (1965). Pain mechanisms: A new theory. *Science, 150*(3699), 971–979. https://doi.org/10.1126/science.150.3699.971
6. Placebo Studies. (2012). Placebo effects on pain: A meta-analysis. *Pain Journal, 152*(1), 23–30. https://doi.org/10.1016/j.pain.2010.11.012
7. Siegel, D. J. (2012). *The developing mind: How relationships and the brain interact to shape who we are* (2nd ed.). Guilford Press.

CHAPTER SEVENTEEN

1. Crum, A. J., Salovey, P., & Achor, S. (2013). Rethinking stress: The role of mindsets in determining the stress response. *Journal of Personality and Social Psychology, 104*(4), 716–733. https://doi.org/10.1037/a0031201
2. Henningsen, P., Zipfel, S., & Herzog, W. (2007). Management of functional somatic syndromes. *The Lancet, 369*(9565), 946–955. https://doi.org/10.1016/S0140-6736(07)60159-7
3. Kabat-Zinn, J. (1990). *Full catastrophe living: Using the wisdom of your body and mind to face stress, pain, and illness.* Delta.
4. LeDoux, J. E. (2000). Emotion circuits in the brain. *Annual Review of Neuroscience, 23*(1), 155–184. https://doi.org/10.1146/annurev.neuro.23.1.155
5. Melzack, R., & Wall, P. D. (1965). Pain mechanisms: A new theory. *Science, 150*(3699), 971–979. https://doi.org/10.1126/science.150.3699.971

6. Placebo Studies. (2012). Placebo effects on pain: A meta-analysis. *Pain Journal, 152*(1), 23–30. https://doi.org/10.1016/j.pain.2010.11.012
7. Siegel, D. J. (2012). *The developing mind: How relationships and the brain interact to shape who we are* (2nd ed.). Guilford Press.
8. Taylor, S. E. (2006). Tend and befriend: Biobehavioral bases of affiliation under stress. *Current Directions in Psychological Science, 15*(6), 273–277. https://doi.org/10.1111/j.1467-8721.2006.00451.x
9. Varela, F. J., Thompson, E., & Rosch, E. (1992). *The embodied mind: Cognitive science and human experience.* MIT Press.
10. Wager, T. D., & Atlas, L. Y. (2015). The neuroscience of placebo effects: Connecting context, learning and health. *Nature Reviews Neuroscience, 16*(7), 403–418. https://doi.org/10.1038/nrn3916

ABOUT DR. SAHAR SWIDAN

DR. SAHAR SWIDAN, PHARMD, RPH, ABAAHP, FAARFM, FMNM, FACA

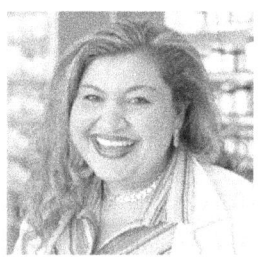

Dr. Swidan is a world-renowned clinical pharmacist, educator, and visionary in integrative pain management and neuroendocrine health. As President and CEO of NeuroPharm and founder of Sahar Skin Care. She brings a rare combination of pharmaceutical precision, functional medicine insight, and entrepreneurial innovation to everything she touches.

A Doctor of Pharmacy with a postdoctoral fellowship in Bio-Pharmaceutics and Gastroenterology from the University of Michigan, Dr. Swidan is also board certified and an advanced fellow in anti-aging and regenerative medicine. She has served on the faculty of University of Michigan, George Washington University School of Medicine and Wayne State University College of Pharmacy, where she has trained thousands of clinicians in the science—and art—of healing.

Internationally sought after for her groundbreaking work in hormone therapy, complex pain syndromes, and personalized therapeutics, she is also co-editor of *Advanced Therapeutics in Pain Medicine* and a key contributor to *Metabolic Therapies in Orthopedics*. Whether she's lecturing on the global stage or guiding patients toward transformation, Dr. Swidan's mission remains the same: to radically shift how we think about pain, aging, and the power of cellular restoration.

ABOUT DR. MATTHEW BENNNETT

DR. MATTHEW BENNETT, MD, FAAOS, ABAARM, FAAMM

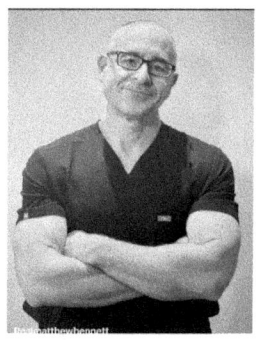

Dr. Matthew Bennett is an orthopedic spine surgeon and functional medicine expert who has dedicated his career to helping individuals overcome chronic pain and unlock their highest potential. With a foundation in Nutritional Sciences from Cornell University, fellowship training at the renowned Texas Back Institute, and dual board certifications in orthopedic surgery and regenerative medicine, Dr. Bennett brings a rare and powerful blend of clinical expertise to his work.

He is the co-editor of *Advanced Therapeutics in Pain Medicine* and has authored multiple book chapters and peer-reviewed research articles in the fields of pain, orthopedics, and spine care. Drawing from both cutting-edge science and personal experience with injury and recovery, he has pioneered a new model of pain care—one that fuses medicine, movement, and mindset.

Through his work at TranscendMed, Dr. Bennett empowers patients to break free from the limitations of chronic pain, cultivate resilience, and reclaim lives of clarity, vitality, and performance.

www.ingramcontent.com/pod-product-compliance
Lightning Source LLC
Chambersburg PA
CBHW060450030426
42337CB00015B/1533